Tympanoplasty, Mastoidectomy, and Stapes Surgery

Ugo Fisch

in collaboration with John May

140 illustrations by Ugo Fisch and Ivan Glitsch
36 tables

1994
Georg Thieme Verlag   Thieme Medical Publishers, Inc.
Stuttgart · New York   New York

Ugo Fisch, M.D.
Professor and Head
ENT Department
University Hospital
8091 Zürich
Switzerland

John May, M.D.
300 South Hawthorne Road
Winston Salem, NC 27103
USA

Library of Congress Cataloging-in-Publication Data

Fisch, Ugo,
   Tympanoplasty, mastoidectomy, and stapes
surgery / Ugo Fisch in collaboration with John
May ; 140 illustrations by Ugo Fisch and Ivan
Glitsch.
     p. cm.
   Includes bibliographical references and index.
   ISBN 3-13-137701-1 (G. Thieme Verlag). --
ISBN 0-86577-559-1 (Thieme Medical Publishers)
   1. Tympanoplasty--Handbooks, manuals, etc.
2. Mastoidectomy--Handbooks, manuals, etc.
3. Myringoplasty--Handbooks, manuals etc.
4. Stapes--Surgery--Handbooks, manuals, etc.
I. May, John, 1955- II. Title.
   [DNLM: 1. Tympanoplasty--methods. 2. Myrin-
goplasty--methods. 3. Mastoid--surgery. 4. Stapes
Surgery--methods. WV 225 F528t 1994]
RF220.F54 1994
617.8'4059--dc20
DNLM/DLC
for Library of Congress   94-20977
              CIP

Important Note: Medicine is an ever-changing science undergoing continual development. Research and clinical experience are continually expanding our knowledge, in particular our knowledge of proper treatment and drug therapy. Insofar as this book mentions any dosage or application, readers may rest assured that the authors, editors and publishers have made every effort to ensure that such references are in accordance with the state of knowledge at the time of production of the book.

Nevertheless this does not involve, imply, or express any guarantee or responsibility on the part of the publishers in respect of any dosage instructions and forms of application stated in the book. Every user is requested to examine carefully the manufacturers' leaflets accompanying each drug and to check, if necessary in consultation with a physician or specialist, whether the dosage schedules mentioned therein or the contraindications stated by the manufacturers differ from the statements made in the present book. Such examination is particularly important with drugs that are either rarely used or have been newly released on the market. Every dosage schedule or every form of application used is entirely at the user's own risk and responsibility. The authors and publishers request every user to report to the publishers any discrepancies or inaccuracies noticed.

Cover drawing by Renate Stockinger

© 1994 Georg Thieme Verlag,
Rüdigerstraße 14, D-70469 Stuttgart, Germany
Thieme Medical Publishers, Inc., 381 Park Avenue
South, New York, N.Y. 10016

Typesetting by Druckhaus Götz GmbH,
D-71636 Ludwigsburg
(CCS-Textline [Linotronic 630])
Printed in Germany by Druckhaus Götz GmbH

ISBN 3-13-137701-1 (GTV, Stuttgart)
ISBN 0-86577-559-1 (TMP, New York)

1 2 3 4 5 6

To Monica
and
to My Teachers

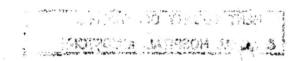

Preface

Every surgical move should be, as in a chess-game, the result of a logical plan. Surgical disasters are usually the consequence of ill-conceived and therefore hazardous actions. Only the constant use of reasonable and logic principles based on knowledge and experience will allow the surgeon to react adequately, even when facing the most unexpected situation.

The aim of this book is to convey a logical approach to the most common problems in otologic surgery. To realize this purpose we have not reviewed all available techniques of tympanoplasty, mastoidectomy, and stapes surgery, but only considered those that have proven of value during 30 years of otologic practice and teaching. Particular care has been taken to explain the reasons determining the choice of a particular technique. Revision surgery, which is the natural harvest of prolonged activity in the otologic field, offered sufficient opportunity to assess the validity of the surgical principles illustrated in this book. Adequate exposure remains the main prerequisite for successful surgery. Most failures of myringoplasty are the consequence of inadequate canalplasty. Wet open cavities are usually the result of insufficient exteriorization. Failures in stapes surgery often derive from limited exposure through a narrow external auditory canal. To achieve adequate exposure, one must be prepared to enlarge a microsurgical keyhole rather than to use inadequately small keys.

The joint preventive efforts of pediatricians and ENT specialists have reduced, in developed countries, the number of patients in need of otologic surgery. The corresponding dilution of surgical expertise has increased the need for simple and reliable otologic techniques. We prefer the endaural approach to the transcanal use of the ear speculum because it provides a larger exposure and allows the use of both hands for ossicular reconstruction and stapes surgery. In view of the reduced opportunities for surgical experience, residents and practicing otologists should also learn to accept their limitations. One should be prepared to refer rare and complex pathologies to those with greater experience and to step out in due time from too difficult surgical adventures to avoid disaster.

The danger of a surgical manual is that it may give a false impression of simplicity and ease. This is why we have attached great importance to the meticulous description of each surgical step. The illustrations in this manual were made by the author and are intended to convey essential surgical features rather than to be a realistic reproduction of a given anatomical situation.

Of course, the manual skills required to perform safe surgery can only be acquired by temporal bone dissection in the laboratory and by carefully supervised surgery in the operating room. Only in this way can one learn to perform an adequate canalplasty reducing the overhang of the anterior canal wall without breaking into the temporomandibular joint, to safely skeletonize the semicircular canals and the tympanomastoid segments of the fallopian canal for the correct exenteration and exteriorization of the retro-

and supralabyrinthine pneumatic spaces, and to perform the steps of stapes surgery with sufficient delicacy of touch. We have tried to make the reader aware of these difficulties throughout the book, particularly in the "rules and hints" sections following each chapter.

A book like this is the result of the effort of many people. I am very greatful to my wife, Monica, for having gracefully accepted that many weekends and vacations were absorbed by the preparation of this book. Sincere thanks go to Mrs. Ch. Hofmann for the invaluable help in typing the manuscript, to Mrs. B. Schmugge for the precious computer instructions, and to Mrs. A. Rapold for trying the impossible and giving me time to write this book within my endless working schedule. I also have to acknowledge the invaluable and dedicated help of Mrs. R. Brandstätter and Mrs. E. Haukenfrers in the operating room, and in compiling the list of instruments cited in this book. My special gratitude goes to Mr. I. Glitsch, who has agreed to give his unique professional touch to the illustrations in spite of his well-deserved retirement and to Dr. John May who, after spending a year of fellowship with us, has taken the trouble to revise the manuscript and to offer many suggestions for its improvement. My thanks also go to Dr. R. Zane, Houston, for his help in correcting the galley proofs. Finally I have to acknowledge the great help of Mr. Menge, Mr. Schäfer, and Ms. Solaro of Thieme, who have used all their expertise to put this book in the proper printed shape.

It is my hope that this manual will help residents find a reliable way through the complex and fascinating world of otologic surgery and be of value to the ENT practitioners in solving some of their challenging daily problems.

Zürich, Spring 1994   U. Fisch

Contents

Chapter 3

Ossiculoplasty   43

Chapter 4

Special Applications with Tympanoplasty   119

Chapter 5

Mastoidectomy   145

Chapter 6

Special Applications of Mastoidectomy   199

Chapter 1
Tympanoplasty

General Considerations

1. Definitions

The surgical reconstruction of the tympano-ossicular system (*tympanoplasty*) includes: *canalplasty*, *myringoplasty*, and *ossiculoplasty*.

Myringoplasty is a technique for reconstructing a vibrating tympanic membrane. The widening of the external auditory canal (canalplasty) is an integral part of myringoplasty. It should be carried out for the grafting of all anterior perforations of the tympanic membrane because it gives the necessary surgical access for their adequate repair. Canalplasty also facilitates healing, cleansing, and second-stage ossiculoplasty. Different types of ossiculoplasty are necessary to restore the sound transmission from the drum to the inner ear.

2. Aims of Tympanoplasty

- Eradication of disease
- Restoration of tympanic aeration
- Reconstruction of a sound-transformer mechanism
- Creation of a dry, self-cleansing cavity

3. Preoperative Care

3.1 Preoperative Investigations

Tubal function. The function of the eustachian tube is assumed to be normal when the Valsalva or Toynbee maneuver is positive.

Tympanometry is performed if the above-mentioned test results are negative.

Knowledge of eustachian tube function is important for proper surgical planning and to assess the chance of a possible hearing improvement. Negative tubal tests, however, are not an absolute contraindication for tympanoplasty. Normal ventilation may indeed be restored in spite of a negative tubal test by surgical excision of scar tissue occluding the tympanic ostium of the eustachian tube. Good aeration of the opposite ear may serve as an indicator of good tubal function.

Temporary closure of perforation. Applying a disk of wet Gelfilm over the remaining drum permits temporary closure of a perforation. Resulting changes in hearing permit assessment of the condition of the ossicular chain and/or the oval and round windows.

Fistula test. The fistula test should always be performed when a patient complains of vertigo or in the presence of a cholesteatoma. It is the unexpected fistula that leads to deafness at surgery. Be certain to maintain a good seal when performing the fistula test to avoid a caloric response to cold air.

3.2 Rules for Preoperative Treatment

The operating microscope or equivalent magnification as well as aspirating tubes is an essential prerequisite for proper preoperative evaluation and treatment. *The aim is to operate, if possible, on a dry, well-ventilated ear.*

- Clean the external canal using *aspiration* to remove fluid, and 3% hydrogen peroxide (H_2O_2) to mollify dry secretion.
- *Apply antibiotic ear drops or ointment on a strip of 0.5-cm ribbon gauze.* The gauze should not be impregnated with too much ointment. The purpose of introducing gauze into the external auditory canal is:
  1) to avoid free diffusion of ototoxic drugs into the middle ear, and
  2) to absorb secretion from the external canal.
  The strip of gauze should be changed *frequently* until it remains dry.

  Avoid:
  1) systemic antibiotics, if there are no signs of general infection,
  2) the use of free ear drops since in the presence of a perforated drum, a sensorineural deafness may be induced.
- If the ear does not become dry after 3 to 4 weeks of treatment, *surgery must be performed in spite of the draining ear.*

3.3 Antibiotic Treatment

Dry ears. Routine perioperative i.v. antibiotic treatment, Bactrim* (trimethoprim sulfamethoxazole) or Augmentin** (amoxicillin and clavulanic acid) is given for myringoplasty, tympanoplasty with extensive bone

work (mastoidectomy, epitympanectomy, posterior tympanotomy, modified radical operation, and reconstruction of an open cavity).

No antibiotics are given for reconstruction of the ossicular chain when the drum is intact (particularly in second-stage operations) as well as for stapedectomy and stapedotomy.

Draining ears. If the preoperative treatment did not succeed in drying the ear, a bacteriologic investigation of the persisting secretion is performed only when the secretion is purulent.

A predominantly clear mucous secretion is related to hyperplastic changes of the mucosa of the tympanic cavity and does not require bacteriologic investigation. Gramnegative microbes such as *Pseudomonas pyocyanea* and *Proteus mirabilis* , as well as fungi, are commonly found in most middle ear secretions because of a superinfection originating from the external canal. If the secretion is not frankly purulent, these microbes do not need specific treatment.

3.4 Preoperative Preparation

The hair is shaved above and behind the ear, (2 cm for tympanoplasty and mastoidectomy). No hair is removed for the endaural approach (stapedotomy, stapedectomy, or second-stage ossicular reconstruction).

The external canal is cleaned by the surgeon a day before. When a perforation is present, the canal is filled with sterile gauze during the surgical preparation to avoid injury to the middle ear by the disinfecting agent. The skin of the operating field and the pinna are cleaned with soap and water and a disinfection solution (Braunol 2000*). No effort is made to disinfect the external canal because we do not believe that sterilization is possible.

---

*   Supplier Hoffmann–La Roche A.G., Basel, Switzerland
** Supplier Beecham

* Polyvinylpyrrolidon – Jodine Compound (Braun Medical AG), Germany

4. Postoperative Care

The operating microscope or equivalent magnification, as well as aspirating tubes, speculum, and forceps are essential pre-requisites for proper postoperative treatment.

4.1 Myringoplasty, Tympanoplasty

- If packing remains dry: nothing for 8–10 days.
- If packing becomes wet: aspirate excess fluid daily from the packing for 6–8 days. The packing is removed under the micro-scope after 6–10 days. Gelfoam pledgets filling the canal are removed by gentle aspiration. Gelfoam pledgets over the fas-cia are left in place for another week. Strips of gauze slightly impregnated with antibi-otic ointment (Terracortril, Pfizer Inter-national, New York) are placed in the canal during this time. Later on, drying strips of gauze impregnated with antibiotic solu-tion (Otosporin, Wellcome Foundation Ltd., London) are used.
- Transmastoid drain, see page 106.

4.2 Open Cavity (Radical Mastoido-Epitympanectomy with Tympanoplasty [Rad. MET])

- Aspirate excess fluid from the packing daily for 6–8 days.
- Remove strips of gauze impregnated with ointment in 3–4 steps at 2–3-day intervals.
- Begin to suction away gelfoam filling the cavity, after 2–3 weeks.
- Use strips of gauze impregnated with oint-ment until granulation tissue has covered the bare bone. Drying gauze with antibi-otic solution is used thereafter.
- Do not forget that in the presence of long-standing preoperative infections, an open cavity may need 1.5–2 months to epithe-lize completely.
- Do not forget that the postoperative treat-ment is as important as the operation itself.

5. Anesthesia

5.1 Local Anesthesia

Indication

Local anesthesia (LA) is used whenever no ex-tensive bone work is needed in combination with an endaural approach (myringoplasty, second-stage ossicular chain reconstruction, stapes surgery).

Premedication

For adults of average weight (70 kg), 10 mg Valium (diazepam) or, if an anxiolytic is required, Dormicum (midazolam) per os 45 minutes before surgery.

Injection

20 ml 1% lidocaine with 2 drops of 1:1,000 epinephrine (final concentration 1:200 000 epinephrine); 5–10 ml thereof are injected as demonstrated in Fig. 1.

The advantage of this method of local an-esthesia is that it causes minimal pain to the patients. Infiltration of the soft tissues sur-rounding the auricle may induce a transient homolateral facial palsy. A study carried out by J. M. Lancer* has shown that no adverse ef-fects were observed either as a consequence of local anesthesia itself, or of the transient fa-

* Lancer, J. M., Fisch, U., Clin. Otolaryngol. 1988; 13:367–374.

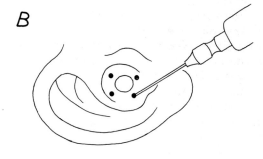

Fig. 1 A

Initial site of injection for local anesthesia

Initially the needle is inserted in the postauricular sulcus and advanced anteroinferiorly. Five ml LA are administered by continuous infiltration during slow withdrawal to block the great auricular nerve. The needle is redirected through the same injection site and advanced anterosuperiorly. An additional 5 ml is given with the aim of blocking the auricular branches of the auriculotemporal nerve.

Fig. 1 B

Canal injections for local anesthesia

Prior to the administration of LA, each patient is warned that there may be some pain or discomfort and that there is the possibility of transient facial weakness for 1–2 hours following injection. The postauricular injection reduces the initial pain, gives an excellent "adequacy of anesthesia" score, and abolishes the unpleasant sensation caused by manipulation of the chorda tympani during surgery.

cial weakness. Both the patient and the surgeon were happy with the quality of the anesthesia.

5.2 General Anesthesia

Premedication

For adults of average weight (70 kg), 10 mg Valium (sedative) or Dolantin (meperidine)-atropine i.m. 30 minutes before surgery.

Induction

Thiopental, etomidate or propofol and fentanyl (0.5 mg). Muscle relaxation with Celocurin. Intubation.

Continuation

Atracurium or Pavulon for muscle relaxation. Artificial respiration with oxygen-nitrous oxide. Repeated injections of fentanyl or alfentanil. Regulation of depth of narcosis with enflurane or isoflurane.

The combination of Valium and fentanyl for general anesthesia avoids

1) the annoying *capillary vasodilation* pro duced by most other anesthetics, and
2) *sensitization of the cardiac conductive system to epinephrine* (as observed, e.g. with Fluothane).

6. Facial Nerve Monitoring

Monitoring facial nerve function using EMG needles placed in the muscles of the face is essential in surgical procedures that carry a risk for the facial nerve (e.g. closed and open mastoido-epitympanectomy, revision surgery after radical mastoidectomy, tympanoplasty in atretic ears). In the past 6 years, we have used the Nicolet system and later on the Xomed NIM-2 system (Fig. 2). Next to the anatomical identification of the position of the facial nerve, the great advantage of monitoring is that constant information on the status of the nerve can be obtained by listening to the spontaneous activity of the facial muscles. There are many occasions in which manipulation carried out away from the facial nerve may lead to a response of the facial muscles indicating that an exposed nerve has been touched inadvertently by the shaft of an instrument, or that granulation thought to be independent is indeed attached to the nerve. Monitoring is utilized in our department for teaching purposes when residents perform open or closed cavity mastoidectomy. Systematic use of facial nerve monitoring in the training of otologic surgeons should reduce and hopefully eliminate the "inevitable" reported rate of 1–3% facial nerve lesions involved in otologic training.

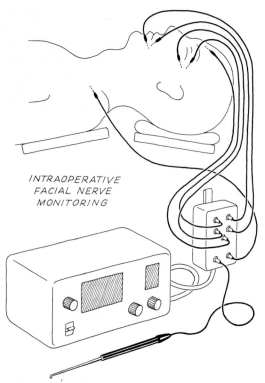

INTRAOPERATIVE
FACIAL NERVE
MONITORING

Fig. 2

Intraoperative facial nerve monitoring.

Position of Electrodes for two channel intraoperative EMG recording with the Xomed-Nerve Integrity monitor (NIM-2). An insulated microraspatory (left and right) is used to assess the position of the facial nerve by electrical stimulation.

7. Instrumentation

(See separate chapter at the end of the book)

8. Rules and Hints

- Communicate with the anesthetist concerning the use of muscle relaxants. Be sure that this information is shared with anesthesia personnel, who may enter the case after it is underway.
- When in doubt about nerve monitor function, it is best to test the nerve at a known location.
- Be sure that the assistants and nurses understand the operation of the monitor so that technical problems are recognized and inadvertent changes are not made to instrument settings.
- Injection of local anesthetics may interfere with the function of the monitor.
- Stimulator probe function can be tested by observing the contractions of an exposed muscle.
- Extreme levels of sound may be generated by aspiration of the ear. The patient should be warned of this prior to beginning. Caution should be used and excessive suctioning near the drum should be avoided because of the risk of acoustic trauma to the inner ear.
- Early in the postoperative period, caution should be used when cleaning the ear to avoid disturbing the graft or the canal flaps.
- Patients should be available for 1 week following stapes surgery, ossiculoplasty, and minor procedures done under local anesthesia. This is necessary for cleaning and maintaining the ear, as well as for reassurance if pain, dizziness, or other symptoms appear.
- After closed or open cavity mastoidoepitympanectomy, patients should be available for 10–14 days, until they can change the ribbon gauze in the canal themselves.
- Flying after stapes surgery and tympanoplasty (ossiculoplasty an myringoplasty) is best avoided for 3 weeks.
- Strict avoidance of water in the ear should be stressed to all patients.
- Patients should be instructed preoperatively of the permanent limitations after ossiculoplasty and stapes surgery (scuba diving, avoidance of intensive manipulations of the external canal with Q-tips, fingers, etc.)

Chapter 2
Myringoplasty

General Considerations

1. Definitions

The term "tympanoplasty" implies reconstruction of the middle ear hearing mechanism with or without tympanic membrane grafting. Grafting of the tympanic membrane is generally called *"myringoplasty"* when the middle ear cavity is not entered and *"tympanoplasty"* when the surgeon works in the middle ear in the presence of an intact ossicular chain. In practice, only small perforations may be closed without extensive work in the middle ear. Therefore, in this atlas, the term *"myringoplasty"* is used for all reconstructions of the tympanic membrane that are not associated with ossiculoplasty. A synonymous term would be "tympanoplasty without reconstruction of the ossicular chain."

2. Surgical Approaches

2.1 Transcanal Approach

With this approach, surgery is performed through an ear speculum in the external canal. The transcanal approach is indicated when the external auditory canal is wide enough to allow complete visualization of a posterior perforation. The approach *cannot* be used when the anterior margin of the perforation is obscured by the overhanging canal wall (Fig. **3 A**).

2.2 Endaural Approach

For this approach, a small incision is made between the tragus and the helix. The entrance of the canal is enlarged with endaural retractors. A posterior overhang of bone can be eliminated with a burr (*broken line*). A more anterior surgical view than with the transcanal approach is achieved. However, most anterior perforations are still obscured by the anteroinferior overhang of the bony external canal (Fig. **3 B**).

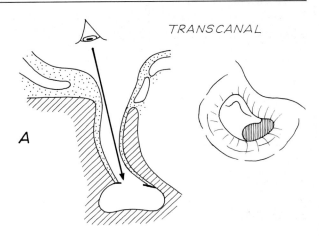

Fig. 3 A

Transcanal approach for myringoplasty

This approach cannot be used for an anterior perforation, which is obscured by the overhanging canal wall.

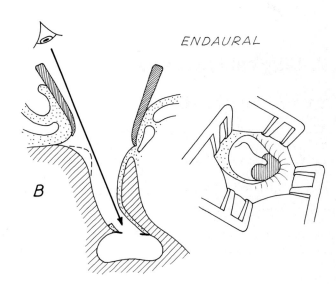

Fig. 3 B

Endaural approach for myringoplasty

A posterior overhang of bone can be eliminated with a burr giving a more anterior surgical view than the transcanal approach. However, most anterior perforations are still obscured by the anteroinferior overhang of the bony external canal.

2.3 Retroauricular Approach

With this approach, the pinna and the attached retroauricular tissues are reflected anteriorly. The removal of the overhanging canal walls (canalplasty, *broken lines*) provides for complete exposure of the anterior edge of the tympanic membrane (Fig. **3 C**).

RETROAURICULAR

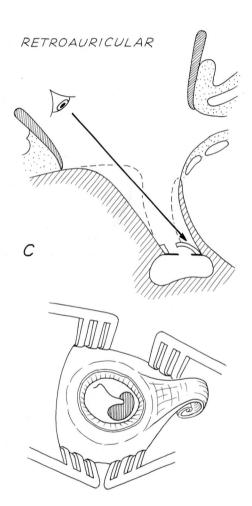

C

Fig. **3 C**

Retroauricular approach for myringoplasty

The retroauricular approach allows a sufficient canalplasty for visualization of all anterior perforations.

3. Selection of Surgical Approach

The *transcanal* approach is mostly used for repairing larger acute traumatic perforations (Fig. **4 A**). The *endaural* approach is selected for posterior perforations (Fig. **4 B**), and the *retroauricular* approach for anterior perforations whose margins cannot be seen entirely through the intact external canal (Fig. **4 C**).

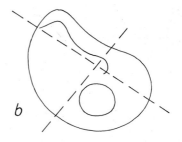

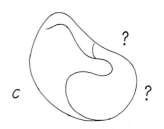

Fig. **4**

Selection of surgical approach for myringoplasty

a: Acute traumatic perforations are repaired through a transcanal approach.
b: Posterior perforations are adequately visualized by an endaural approach.
c: Anterior perforations with margins that cannot be seen entirely through the intact external canal require a retroauricular approach.

4. Grafting Technique

Two principle techniques are used for *grafting the tympanic membrane:*

1. the *anterior underlay,* and
2. the *overlay.*

4.1 Anterior Underlay (Fig. 5)

The presence of an anterior remnant of the tympanic membrane (at least of the fibrous tympanic annulus) is required for this type of fascial graft. The graft is placed *under* the anterior remnant of the tympanic membrane and *over* the posterior tympanic sulcus. With the exception of perforations limited to the anteroinferior quadrant, the graft lies under the malleus handle.

4.2 Overlay (Fig. 6)

This technique is used when there is no remnant of the tympanic membrane. A new bony sulcus is drilled to support the fascia at the lateral opening of the tympanic cavity. The graft rests over the sulcus and underneath the malleus handle. The edges of the graft are covered by meatal skin.

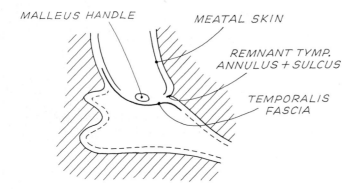

Fig. 5

Anterior underlay of temporalis fascia

The graft is placed *under* the anterior remnant of the tympanic membrane and *over* the posterior tympanic sulcus. The graft lies under the malleus handle.

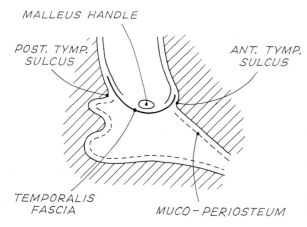

Fig. 6

Overlay of temporalis fascia

The graft rests over the anterior and posterior tympanic sulcus and underneath the malleus handle. The edges of the graft are covered by meatal skin.

Specific Surgical Techniques

1. Transcanal Approach

1.1 Surgical Technique

The transcanal approach is mostly used as an emergency procedure for the repair of large acute traumatic perforations of the tympanic membrane.

1.2 Surgical Highlights

- Local anesthesia
- Use of the ear speculum
- Outfolding of perforation margins
- Intra- and extratympanic fixation of repositioned perforation margins

1.3 Surgical Steps

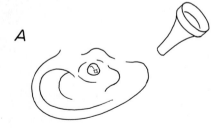

TRANSCANAL APPROACH

Fig. 7 A

Use of the ear speculum

The traumatic perforation is visualized through the ear speculum. No incisions are made in the external auditory canal.

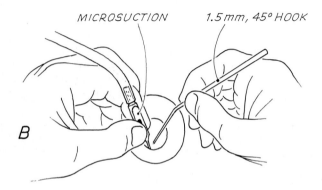

MICROSUCTION   1.5 mm, 45° HOOK

Fig. 7 B

Fixation of the ear speculum

The left hand holds the ear speculum between the index and third finger as well as the microsuction between the thumb and index finger. The right hand carries the instruments needed to reposition the perforation margins (mainly a 1.5-mm, 45° hook).

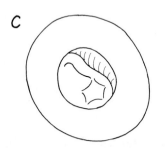

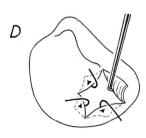

Fig. 7 C

Exposure of the traumatic perforation

Note the infolded edges of the perforation, which has the typical irregular shape.

Fig. 7 D

Outfolding of perforation margins

The edges of the perforation are outfolded using a 1.5-mm, 90° hook.

Fig. 7 **E**

Intratympanic fixation of perforation margins

The outfolded perforation margins are kept in position by intratympanic Gelfoam pledgets soaked in Ringer's solution.

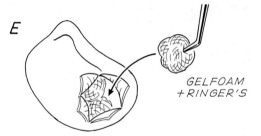

E

GELFOAM
+RINGER'S

Fig. 7 **F**

Intratympanic Gelfoam in place

Surgical site following introduction of the intratympanic Gelfoam pledgets.

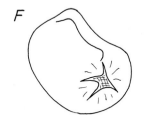

F

Fig. 7 **G**

Extratympanic fixation of perforation margins

A piece of Gelfilm is placed briefly in Ringer's solution and then used to stabilize the outer surface of the lacerated tympanic membrane. The external canal is packed with Gelfoam and Terra-Cortril gauze for 5 to 8 days. Antibiotic coverage (Bactrim, Augmentin) is also given for 5 to 8 days.

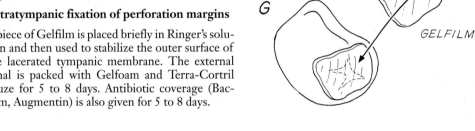

G

GELFILM

For other applications of the transcanal approach see page 120.

2. Endaural Approach

2.1 Surgical Technique

This technique is used for posterior perforations with margins that can be clearly visualized through the external auditory canal.

2.2 Surgical Highlights

- Local anesthesia
- Endaural incision
- Refreshing of perforation margins
- Elevation of tympanomeatal flap
- Anterior fascial underlay
- Fixation of underlaid fascia with intratympanic Gelfoam

2.3 Surgical Steps

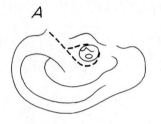

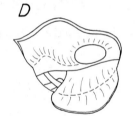

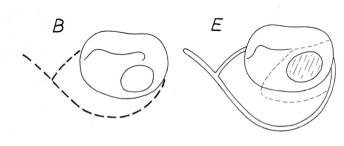

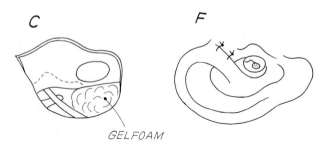

GELFOAM

Fig. **8 A**

Endaural incision

The endaural incision is 5 mm long and is performed between the tragus and the crus helicis.

Fig. **8 B**

Tympanomeatal flap and refreshing of perforation margins

The skin incisions for the tympanomeatal flap are carried from the tympanic annulus at 7 o'clock and 1 o'clock in an ascending spiral fashion to meet the endaural incision. The edges of the perforation are refreshed with biopsy forceps before the tympanomeatal flap is elevated (see also Fig. 11 A).

Fig. **8 C**

Intratympanic Gelfoam

Gelfoam pledgets soaked in Ringer's solution are placed in the hypotympanum following elevation of the tympanomeatal flap. The mobility of the ossicular chain is checked at this stage and found to be intact.

Fig. **8 D**

Anterior underlay of graft

Fresh tragal perichondrium (see also Figs. 59 and 60) is introduced under the perforated drum and over the posterior tympanic sulcus.

Fig. **8 E**

Repositioning the tympanomeatal flap

The tympanomeatal flap is placed back in its original position and secured with small pledgets of Gelfoam. The broken line shows the extent of the underlaid tragal perichondrium.

Fig. **8 F**

Wound closure

Two 3:0 Ethibond sutures are used to close the endaural incision.

3. Retroauricular Approach

3.1 Surgical Technique

The retroauricular approach is mainly used for anterior perforations with margins that are obscured by the overhanging canal wall. In most instances a **canalplasty** is an integral part of the procedure. The elevation of a *meatal skin flap* is a prerequisite for achieving an adequate canalplasty.

3.2 Surgical Highlights

- General anesthesia
- Retroauricular skin incision
- Meatal skin flap
- Canalplasty
- Anterior underlay or overlay grafting
- Antrotomy and epitympanotomy (if needed)

3.3 Surgical Steps

Fig. **9 A**

Skin incision

The retroauricular skin incision is carried out along the hairline and is made only through skin, preserving the underlying fascia and periostium.

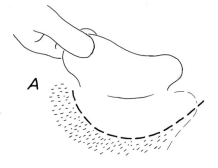

Fig. **9 B**

Periosteal flap

Following elevation of the skin, a retroauricular periosteal flap is formed. This flap will be repositioned and sutured to the surrounding soft tissues at the end of surgery. The periosteal flap may also be used to cover the posterior surface of the canal wall when a mastoidectomy is performed (see Fig. 80 G).

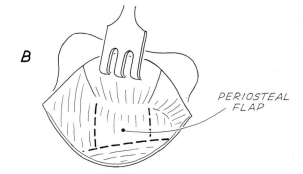

PERIOSTEAL FLAP

Fig. **9 C**

Exposure of the external auditory canal

The periosteal flap is elevated from the bone with a mastoid raspatory. The posterior limb of the canal incision (*A–B*) is carried out with a No. 15 blade, remaining a few millimeters deeper than the entrance of the bony external canal.

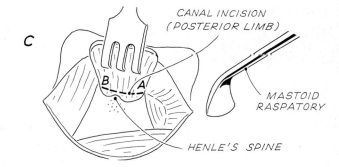

CANAL INCISION (POSTERIOR LIMB)

MASTOID RASPATORY

HENLE'S SPINE

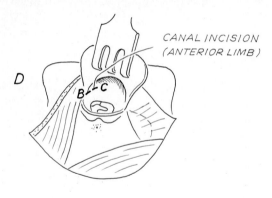

CANAL INCISION
(ANTERIOR LIMB)

D

B—C

Fig. **9 D**

Exposure of the external auditory canal (cont.)

The external auditory canal is opened and the canal incision extended along the anterior meatal wall (*B–C*).

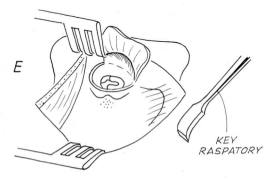

E

KEY
RASPATORY

Fig. **9 E**

Exposure of the external auditory canal (cont.)

The lateral canal skin is elevated with a Key raspatory. A superior articulated retroauricular retractor is introduced.

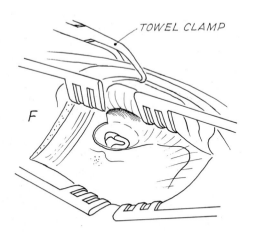

TOWEL CLAMP

F

Fig. **9 F**

Exposure of the mastoid

A second, inferior retroauricular retractor achieves the exposure of the mastoid plane from the mastoid tip to the temporal line. The retroauricular soft tissues attached to the pinna are held anteriorly with a towel clamp.

Meatal Skin Flap

Fig. 9 G

Meatal skin flap

The meatal skin is incised, forming an anterior ascending spire (D–C). Care should be taken to remain with the tip of the No. 11 blade (scalpel handle No. 4) on the bone of the canal wall.

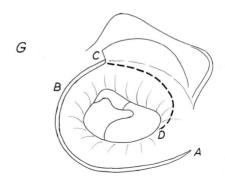

Fig. 9 H

Meatal skin flap (cont.)

The meatal skin is elevated from the bone by means of a "universal" microdissector. The elevation of the skin is carried out under direct vision until the posterosuperior margin of the drum and the anteroinferior overhang of canal bone are exposed.

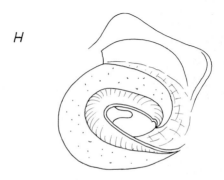

Fig. 9 I

Meatal skin flap (cont.)

The elevated meatal skin is cut medially with straight and curved tympanoplasty microscissors in a circular fashion (D-E) remaining 2 mm lateral from the posterosuperior tympanic annulus and on the anteroinferior edge of the overhanging canal bone. In this way, the lateral meatal skin is separated from the medial sleeve of meatal skin still attached to the annulus.

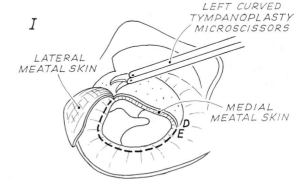

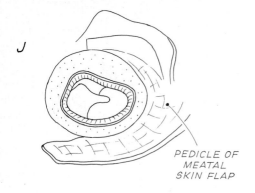

J

PEDICLE OF
MEATAL
SKIN FLAP

Fig. 9 J

Meatal skin flap (cont.)

The inferiorly based meatal skin flap is elevated out of the external canal.

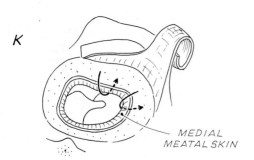

K

MEDIAL
MEATAL SKIN

Fig. 9 K

Meatal skin flap (cont.)

Surgical site following elevation of the meatal skin flap showing the overhanging bony canal wall (*arrows*).

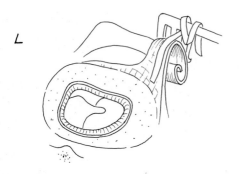

L

Fig. 9 L

Meatal skin flap (cont.)

The lateral meatal skin flap is kept away from the operative field by a small malleable strip of aluminum anchored to the retroauricular wound retractor.

Canalplasty

Fig. 9 M

Canalplasty

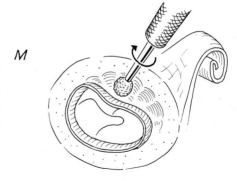

M

The external bony canal is enlarged with sharp and diamond burrs, eliminating all bone overhangs, particularly anterior and inferior. Care is taken to avoid breaking into the temporomandibular joint anteriorly. A bluish pink discoloration of the last layer of bone indicates the position of the TM joint if irrigation is used while drilling.

Fig. 9 N

Canalplasty (cont.)

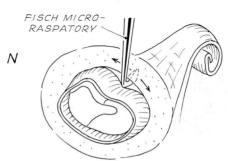

FISCH MICRO-
RASPATORY

N

The overhanging canal bone is removed in steps to provide for elevation of the meatal skin before drilling away the overlying bone.

Fig. 9 O

Canalplasty (cont.)

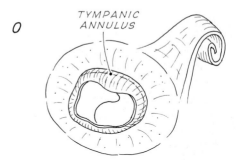

TYMPANIC
ANNULUS

O

When the canalplasty is completed, the entire tympanic annulus is visible with one position of the microscope. After canalplasty, the shape of the external canal corresponds to that of an inverted truncated cone with an outer diameter that is nearly twice that of the tympanic membrane.

Fig. 9 P

Canalplasty (cont.)

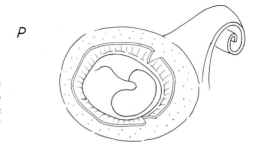

P

The medial canal skin is repositioned against the enlarged bony canal wall, exposing the entire tympanic annulus. All margins of the perforation are clearly visible. Sometimes relaxing incisions may be necessary.

Grafting of Tympanic Membrane

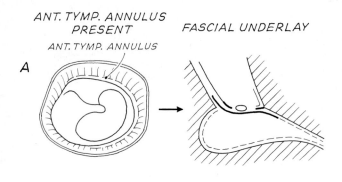

ANT. TYMP. ANNULUS
PRESENT

ANT. TYMP. ANNULUS

A

FASCIAL UNDERLAY

Fig. 10

Indications for anterior underlay and overlay grafting

A Anterior underlay grafting is indicated when the anterior margin of the tympanic membrane or at least the anterior tympanic annulus is present. The graft lies *under* the anterior remnant of the tympanic membrane and *over* the posterior sulcus of tympanic bone.

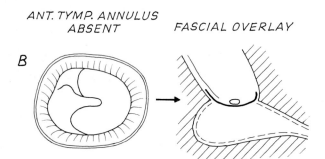

ANT. TYMP. ANNULUS
ABSENT

B

FASCIAL OVERLAY

B The overlay grafting technique is chosen when there is no remnant of the tympanic membrane (see also Fig. 6, p. 14). The overlaid graft rests circumferentially *over* the bony tympanic sulcus.

Anterior Fascial Underlay

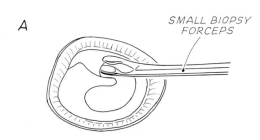

A

SMALL BIOPSY
FORCEPS

Fig. 11 A

Refreshing the perforation margins

The margin of the perforation is refreshed with small biopsy forceps before elevation of the tympanomeatal flap, to provide sufficient stability of the drum.

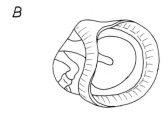

B

Fig. 11 B

Elevation of the tympanomeatal flap and inspection of the ossicular chain

A posterosuperior tympanomeatal flap is elevated, exposing the malleus neck, the long process of the incus, and the stapes head.

Fig. 11 C

Separation of the incudostapedial joint

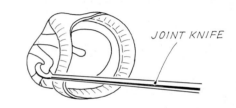

JOINT KNIFE

The incudostapedial joint is separated by means of a joint knife to avoid injury of the inner ear when manipulating along the malleus handle. No special measures are taken at the end of the procedure to readapt the incudostapedial joint. If the lenticular process remains intact, the natural reapproximation of the joint ensures full functional recovery. The mobility of the ossicular chain is best assessed at this stage.

Fig. 12

Preservation of the anterior tympanomeatal angle

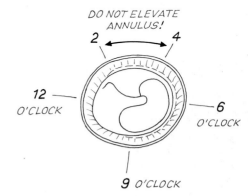

DO NOT ELEVATE ANNULUS!

2 ← → 4

12 O'CLOCK

6 O'CLOCK

9 O'CLOCK

The tympanic annulus should *never* be elevated between 2 o'clock and 4 o'clock on the right side (8–10 o'clock on the left side) because an intact anterior tympanomeatal angle is essential for optimal functional end results. Violation of the anterior "sacred" attachment of the annulus induces blunting of the tympanomeatal angle and lateralization of the drum. This reduces the vibratory properties of the drum.

Sites of Support for the Underlay Graft

The fixation of the underlaid graft varies according the size and position of the perforation (anteroinferior, anterosuperior, or subtotal).

Fig. 13 A

Underlay grafting for anteroinferior perforation

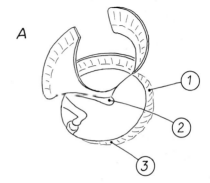

A perforation limited to the anteroinferior quadrant of the drum permits elevation of the inferior tympanomeatal flap until the upper edge of the perforation is reached (4 o'clock). The epithelium covering the tip of the malleus is elevated a few millimeters, exposing the underlying bone. In this case, the fixation of the underlaid fascia can be obtained by placing it

1. over the anteroinferior tympanic sulcus,
2. over the bared tip of the malleus handle, and
3. over the posterior tympanic sulcus.

In anteroinferior perforations there is no need for intratympanic Gelfoam to support the graft anteriorly. This helps to avoid possible obstruction of the eustachian tube in the postoperative period.

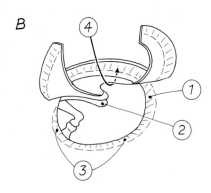

Fig. 13 B

Underlay grafting for anterosuperior perforation (first alternative)

Perforations reaching the anterosuperior quadrant of the drum require special anterior support. Pledgets of Gelfoam soaked in Ringer's solution introduced in the anterior tympanic cavity may support the graft against the undersurface of the drum and tympanic sulcus. In this situation, the underlaid graft is supported

1. on the inferior tympanic sulcus,
2. under the tip of the malleus handle,
3. on the posterior tympanic sulcus, and
4. at the anterior undersurface of the tympanic membrane and adjacent bone.

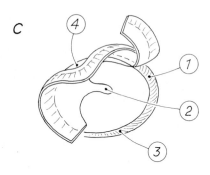

Fig. 13 C

Underlaying grafting for anterosuperior perforation (second alternative)

Effective fixation of the underlay graft in extensive anterosuperior perforations is obtained by detaching the tympanic annulus from the sulcus at 1 o'clock (11 o'clock for the left side) and by pulling the upper edge of the fascia through the resulting gap between the annulus and sulcus. In this situation, the graft is supported

1. on the inferior tympanic sulcus,
2. under the malleus handle,
3. on the posterior tympanic sulcus, and
4. between the anterosuperior tympanic annulus and sulcus.

The anterosuperior fixation of the fascia avoids postoperative obstruction by Gelfoam placed close to tympanic ostium of the eustachian tube.

Fig. 13 D

Underlay grafting for subtotal perforation

In subtotal perforations, only a limited anterior remnant of the tympanic membrane is present. In this situation, the underlaid fascia can only be supported by means of Gelfoam pledgets soaked in Ringer's solution. The anterior annulus should not be separated for pulling through the fascia because this would compromise the stability of the anterior tympanomeatal angle (see Fig. 12). In subtotal perforations, the underlaid graft is supported

1. on the inferior tympanic sulcus,
2. under the malleus handle,
3. on the posterior tympanic sulcus,
4. on the incisura rivini, and
5. at the undersurface of the anterior tympanic remnant with adjacent bone.

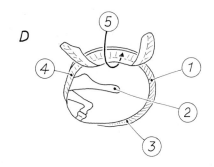

Underlay Grafting for Anteroinferior Perforation

Fig. 14 A

Elevation and division of the tympanomeatal flap

The tympanomeatal flap is elevated posteriorly and divided with straight tympanoplasty microscissors.

Fig. 14 B

Elevation of the tympanomeatal flap (cont.)

The tympanomeatal flaps are elevated anteriorly like swinging doors. The superior flap remains attached to the malleus neck. The inferior flap is separated from the tympanic sulcus up to the cranial edge of the perforation (4 o'clock).

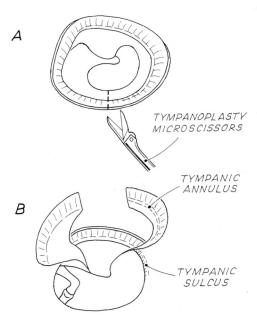

Fig. 14 C

Baring the malleus tip

The tympanic membrane is elevated from the tip of the malleus to avoid burying epidermal rests under it. This maneuver is performed with a 2.5-mm, 45° hook while the malleus is kept lateralized with a 1.5-mm, 45° hook held in the left hand. This results in a separation of the incudostapedial joint (see Fig. 11 C). Care must be taken to avoid elevating the tympanic membrane from the complete malleus handle. This will prevent lateralization of the new tympanic membrane from the malleus handle as it heals.

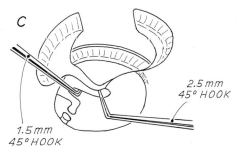

D

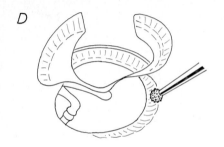

Fig. **14 D**

Drilling a new tympanic sulcus

A new tympanic sulcus is drilled with diamond burrs along the inferoposterior edge of the external auditory canal.

E

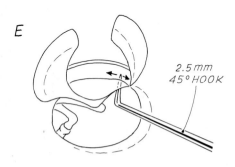

2.5mm
45° HOOK

Fig. **14 E**

Anterior bed for fascial underlay

A raw surface is scraped along the undersurface of the drum and adjacent bone using a 2.5-mm, 45° hook.

F

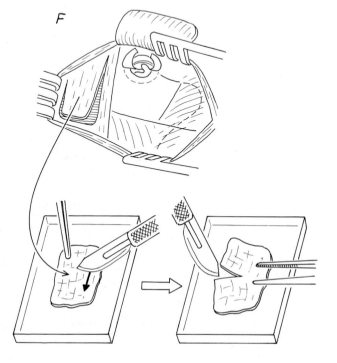

Fig. **14 F**

Harvesting and preparation of the temporalis fascia

The superior retroauricular wound retractor is removed, exposing the temporalis muscle. An incision is made through the fascia 5 mm above the caudal edge of the muscle. The fascia is then separated from the underlying muscle using the flat handle of the knife (No. 7). The desired quantity of fascia is cut out with a pair of curved fascia scissors. The graft is then placed over a glass board, and the excess fat and muscle tissue are removed with a No. 20 blade. An incision is made with the knife according to the expected position of the malleus handle.

Fig. 14 G

Fixation of the underlaid graft

The fascia is kept moist to avoid killing the fibro-cytes, and therefore speed up revascularization and healing. The fresh graft is introduced under the anterior margin of the perforation. Support is provided by the tympanic sulcus (inferior and posterior) and by the bare tip of the malleus handle. There is no need to introduce Gelfoam into the middle ear.

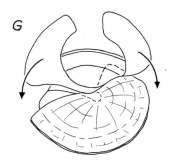

Fig. 14 H

Repositioning the tympanomeatal flaps

The swinging-door tympanomeatal flaps are re-positioned, keeping the fascia locked on the tympanic sulcus.

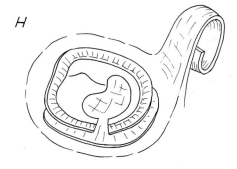

Fig. 14 I

Repositioning the meatal skin flap

The meatal skin flap is placed in its original position covering the posterior edge of the fascia and the posterior canal wall. Gelfoam soaked in Oto-sporin is used to keep the tympanomeatal flaps and the meatal skin in place. Reepithelization of the anterosuperior canal wall requires 3 to 4 weeks.

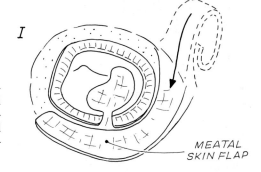

MEATAL SKIN FLAP

Underlay Grafting for Anterosuperior Perforation

a) First Alternative: Intratympanic Gelfoam (see also Fig. 13 B)

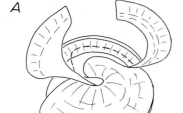

A

Fig. **15 A**

Position of underlaid fascia

For this type of underlay, scraping of the undersurface of the drum and adjacent bone is more extensive than for anteroinferior perforations (see Fig. 14 E). The graft is placed entirely under the malleus handle and rests over the posteroinferior tympanic sulcus.

B

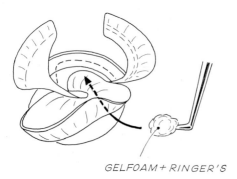

GELFOAM + RINGER'S

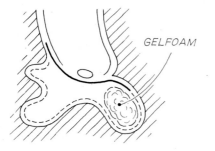

GELFOAM

Fig. **15 B**

Gelfoam for intratympanic fascial support

Gelfoam pledgets soaked in Ringer's solution are introduced into the anterior hypotympanum and protympanum to support the fascia against the raw undersurface of the anterior tympanic membrane and adjacent bone. The disadvantage of this type of anterior support of the graft is the temporary obstruction of the tympanic ostium of the eustachian tube. To facilitate healing, antrotomy with a temporary transmastoid drain is usually associated with this type of underlay grafting (see p. 106).

b) Second Alternative: Anterosuperior Fixation of Graft (see also Fig. **13 C**)

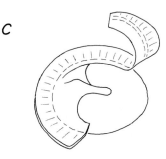

C

Fig. **15 C**

Separation of tympanic annulus from sulcus

The tympanic annulus is separated from the sulcus between 1 o'clock and 2 o'clock.

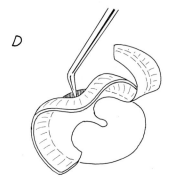

D

Fig. **15 D**

Separation of tympanic annulus from sulcus (cont.)

A 2.5-mm, 45° hook is used to separate the annulus from the tympanic sulcus.

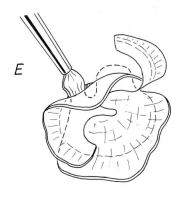

E

Fig. **15 E**

Fixation of fascia

The temporalis fascia is pulled with a microsuction tube through the gap between the tympanic annulus and sulcus.

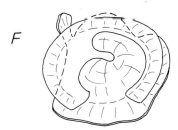

F

Fig. **15 F**

Final position of underlaid fascia

The fascia lies posteriorly and inferiorly on the tympanic sulcus and is kept against the undersurface of the drum and adjacent bone by the anterosuperior fixation between the annulus and sulcus. There is no need for intratympanic Gelfoam, so the problem of temporary occlusion of the tympanic ostium of the eustachian tube is avoided.

Underlay Grafting in Subtotal Perforations
(see also Fig. **13 D**)

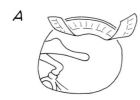

Fig. **16 A**

Surgical site in subtotal perforation

The remnant of the tympanic membrane with surrounding meatal skin is limited to the anterior tympanomeatal angle.

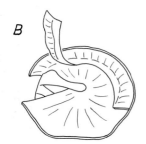

Fig. **16 B**

Position of underlaid temporalis fascia

After scraping the undersurface of the tympanic membrane and adjacent bone, the fascia is placed under the drum and under the malleus handle. Posterior support is given by the tympanic sulcus.

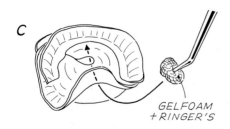

GELFOAM
+ RINGER'S

Fig. **16 C**

Anterior and superior fixation of underlaid fascia

The fascia is supported anteriorly by Gelfoam pledgets soaked in Ringer's solution. Superior fixation is obtained by the overlapping of both cranial limbs of the fascia over the malleus neck.

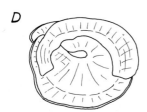

Fig. **16 D**

Final situation of underlaid graft

The malleus tip is situated over the fascia. Both tympanomeatal flaps are replaced, fixing the fascia on the tympanic sulcus.

Overlay Grafting of Tympanic Membrane

Overlay grafting is used in total perforations of the tympanic membrane (no remnant of the annulus present). The temporalis fascia is placed over the circular bony tympanic sulcus (see also Fig. **10 B**, p. 24).

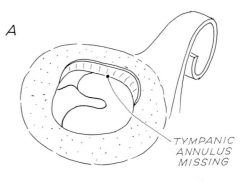

A

Fig. **17 A**

Absence of anterior tympanic annulus

The anterior tympanic annulus is missing. The meatal skin remnant is removed because the indication for a fascial overlay is present.

TYMPANIC ANNULUS MISSING

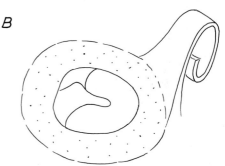

B

Fig. **17 B**

Surgical site following removal of the anterior meatal skin remnant

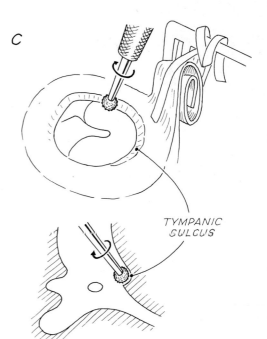

C

Fig. **17 C**

Formation of a new circumferential tympanic sulcus

The meatal skin flap is kept away by a malleable strip of aluminum anchored to the inferior retroauricular retractor. A circumferential tympanic sulcus is drilled with a small diamond burr.

TYMPANIC SULCUS

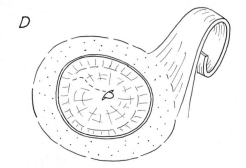

Fig. **17 D**

Anchoring of the overlaid fascia to the malleus tip

Fresh temporalis fascia (see also Fig. 14 F) is used to cover the tympanic cavity as an overlay graft. The tip of the manubrium mallei rests over the fascia through a separate incision. This is an alternative method to that described for fascial fixation in subtotal perforations (see Figs. 16 A, B, C, D).

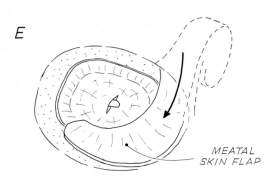

MEATAL
SKIN FLAP

Fig. **17 E**

Repositioning the meatal skin

The meatal skin flap is replaced, covering the inferoposterior overlaid temporalis fascia.

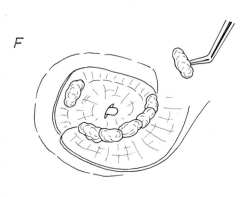

Fig. **17 F**

Fixation of the overlaid fascia

The overlaid fascia, as well as the meatal skin flap, is kept in position by pledgets of Gelfoam soaked in antibiotic solution (Otosporin, Wellcome) placed over the new tympanic sulcus.

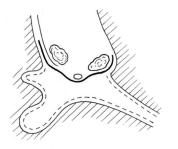

4. Antrotomy

4.1 Surgical Technique

Antrotomy in conjunction with myringo-plasty is carried out when eustachian tube function is questionable or when the middle ear mucosa is abnormal (polypoid or granu-lating).

4.2 Surgical Highlights

- Exposure of the antrum without lowering the entrance of the bony external canal
- Water test for epitympanic patency
- Introduction of a mastoid drain through a separate retroauricular incision

4.3 Surgical Steps

Fig. **18 A**

Identification of the antrum

The position of the antrum is determined by the intersection of two lines parallel to the superior and posterior canal walls.

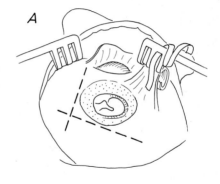

Fig. **18 B**

Antrotomy

The middle cranial fossa dura and the sigmoid sinus are identified through the last shell of bone covering them. The antrum is found by drilling away the bone between the middle cranial fossa dura and the sigmoid sinus. No bone should be removed over the superior and posterior entrance of the external canal. Failure to respect the bone in this area may lead to ingrowth of skin from the external canal into the antrum. The external canal is packed with Gelfoam soaked in Ringer's solution to avoid contamination by bone dust in the middle ear while drilling over the antrum.

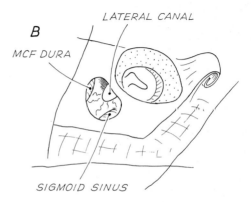

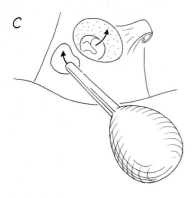

C

Fig. 18 C

Water test for epitympanic patency

Ringer's solution is irrigated into the antrum with a rubber bulb to test whether there is a free communication between antrum and middle ear. If the water test result is positive, there is no need for further exposure of the epitympanum. If the water test result is negative, an *atticotomy* is performed. Reestablishment of the patency of the attic may require removal of pathologic mucosa surrounding the ossicles. Sometimes removal of the incus and malleus head is also required. On rare occasions, a posterior tympanotomy may be necessary to improve the ventilation of the mastoid. If the incus is removed, an incus interposition is performed whenever possible to restore the ossicular chain.

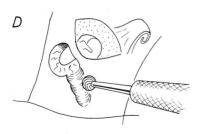

D

Fig. 18 D

Transmastoid drainage of the antrum

After the antrum has been exposed, a groove is drilled in the mastoid bone to accomodate the transmastoid drain (see Fig. 56, p. 106).

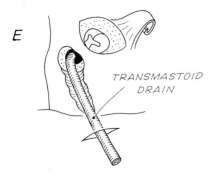

E

TRANSMASTOID
DRAIN

Fig. 18 E

Mastoid drain in place

The transmastoid drain is placed with its bend in the antrum and is led into the bony groove through a separate retroauricular skin incision, using a curved clamp.

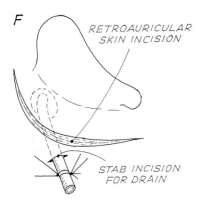

F

RETROAURICULAR
SKIN INCISION

STAB INCISION
FOR DRAIN

Fig. 18 F

Wound closure

The retroauricular skin incision is ready for closure. The mastoid drain is fixed to the skin with a silk suture. Aspiration through the mastoid drain is carried out daily with a smaller diameter suction tube for 2–4 days postoperatively. The patient can perform a Valsalva maneuver 1 day following surgery. The mastoid drain is removed when no secretion is aspirated through it (usually 4 days postoperatively). In patients with tubal dysfunction, the transmastoid drain is left in place for 10–14 days.

5. Complications of Myringoplasty

5.1 Underlay Grafting

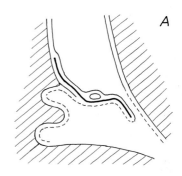

Fig. **19 A**

Anterior reperforation

This complication occurs if underlay grafting is attempted without clear visualization of the anterior tympanic annulus (insufficient canalplasty).

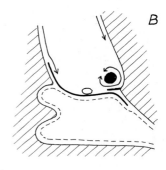

Fig. **19 B**

Anterior tympanomeatal cholesteatoma

This complication results from the infolding of the skin lining of the anterior tympanomeatal angle. The Gelfoam pledgets used to keep the meatal skin in position should be removed within 2 weeks to avoid the formation of an anterior tympanomeatal cholesteatoma.

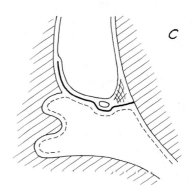

Fig. **19 C**

Blunting the anterior tympanomeatal angle

This complication occurs if the anterior tympanic annulus has been separated from the sulcus (see Fig. 12).

5.2 Overlay Grafting

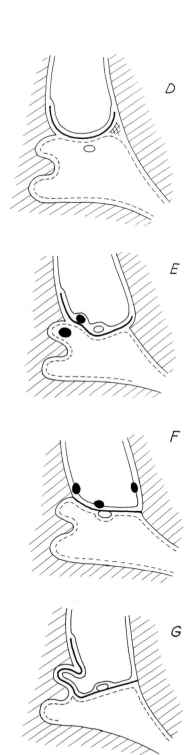

Fig. **19 D**

Lateral displacement of the graft

This complication occurs when no adequate anterior sulcus has been drilled and the overlay graft has not been placed under the malleus handle.

Fig. **19 E**

Inclusion or residual cholesteatoma

Inclusion cholesteatoma is a typical complication of overlaid grafting when the deepithelization of the lateral surface of the drum has not been complete. *Residual* cholesteatoma occurs when remnants of epidermis have been left inside the middle ear cavity. This complication can also occur after underlay grafting.

Fig. **19 F**

Cholesteatoma pearls

Small epidermal cysts may result from irregularities of the epithelization on the outer surface of the graft or on the canal wall. This complication is also possible in underlay grafting.

Fig. **19 G**

Retraction pocket

This complication results from insufficient eustachian tube function. Prevention may be attempted by reinforcing the posterior superior quadrant of the drum with septal cartilage and by introducing Silastic sheeting in the middle ear and the eustachian tube (see pp. 99 and 101).

6. Results

Residents and chief residents in our department operated on 373 patients because of a chronic otitis media with central perforation between 1977 and 1987. The cumulative percentage of perforation closures was of 89% (232/261) at the end of the first postoperative year and 86% (46/53) after 5–15 years (Table 1).

No difference was found in the rate of closure of posterior (86%) and anterior (83%) perforations (Table 2). These results confirm the value of canalplasty for adequate exposure of anterior perforations.

The hearing results of myringoplasty (Table 3) are remarkably stable over 5–15 years postoperative. A closure of the air–bone gap to 0–30 dB was achieved by 85% of the patients at the end of the first postoperative year and by 89% of the patients after 15 years (corresponding preoperative value of 65%). These results show that myringoplasty is a very successful operation, particularly in the presence of an intact ossicular chain.

Table 1 Percentage of perforation closure at long-term follow-up

Follow-up (years)	Perforation Closure	(%)
1	232/261	(89)
5	53/61	(87)
10	46/53	(86)
15	18/21	(86)

Table 2 Rate of perforation closure in relation to localization of the perforation. Anterior: perforation anterior to the malleus handle. Posterior: perforation posterior to the malleus handle. Subtotal: anterior perforation extending posterior to the malleus handle. Note that there is no statistical difference between the rate of closure of the different perforation types (χ^2 test). Results of myringoplasty (5–15-year follow-up = 135)

Localization of Perforation	Rate of Perforation closure	(%)
anterior	54/65	(83)
posterior	30/35	(86)
subtotal	28/35	(80)

Table 3 Pre- and postoperative hearing in 135 patients with myringoplasty for chronic otitis media and intact ossicular chain. The air–bone gap was calculated for the frequencies 0.5, 1, 2 and 4 kHz. Hearing results of myringoplasty (1–15-year follow-up, n = 135)

Air–Bone Gap (dB)	Preop (n = 261)	1 (n = 232)	Follow-up (years) 5 (n = 61)	10 (n = 53)	15 (n = 21)
0–10	9%	38%	33%	41%	44%
0–20	36%	65%	65%	61%	74%
0–30	65%	85%	86%	84%	89%
30	35%	15%	14%	16%	11%

7. Rules and Hints

- Enlarge the bony external canal to the point at which the entire tympanic sulcus can be visualized with one position of the microscope. This facilitates placement of the fascial graft.
- Do not leave bony overhangs of the meatal wall. The postoperative care will be easier, and there will be no problems with self-cleansing of the external canal.
- Create a new anterior tympanic sulcus whenever the anterior fibrous annulus is missing. This prevents blunting of the anterior tympanomeatal angle.
- Disarticulate the incudostapedial joint before carrying out extensive work on the malleus handle. This prevents postoperative sensorineural hearing loss and tinnitus.
- Use transmastoid drainage if preoperative ventilation of the middle ear is insufficient. This will avoid overloading the eustachian tube by performing the double task of clearing the middle ear of accumulated blood and ensuring ventilation.
- Meticulous hemostasis (infiltration with local anesthetic, coagulation with bipolar microforceps) facilitates handling of the grafts and flaps.
- Elevation of the meatal skin flap requires careful attention to preserve its integrity. A wet ribbon gauze should be used to separate the flap from the bone; sharp dissection is necessary at the tympanosquamous suture.
- It is critical to preserve the inferior pedicle of the meatal skin flap when exposing the tympanic ring to ensure adequate vascular supply.
- Gelfoam placed over a defective mucosal lining of the middle ear may cause extensive scarring, compromising the success of subsequent ossicular reconstruction. Therefore, only minimal amounts of Gelfoam should be placed in the middle ear.
- Stage functional surgery if the stapes suprastructure, the malleus handle, or both are missing in large perforations.
- Place a thick Silastic sheet or Gelfilm in the cavum tympani and the eustachian tube in the presence of defective middle ear mucosa.
- Time spent performing an adequate canalplasty is compensated by the time gained by improved exposure during grafting of the tympanic membrane.
- An adequate canalplasty is important for the exposure needed for proper ossiculoplasty.
- One of the causes of a lateralized drum is inaccurate identification of the level of the tympanic sulcus as a result of inadequate canalplasty.
- Use the retroauricular approach in all anterior and subtotal perforations.
- Perform canalplasty in all anterior and subtotal perforations.
- Canalplasty facilitates healing and possible second-stage surgery.
- Stage functional surgery if the stapes suprastructure, the malleus handle, or both are missing in large perforations.
- The fascial graft can be placed over the tip of the malleus only in perforations that do not extend into the anterosuperior portion of the drum.
- Perforations extending into the anterosuperior portion of the drum require fixation of the underlaid fascia between the annulus and sulcus above the "sacred" anterior tympanomeatal angle.
- In overlay grafting, the tip of the malleus is placed through the graft for proper fixation.
- We do not favor deepithelization of the drum with overlay grafting. This is because an anterior underlay is preferable for maintaining the integrity of the anterior tympanomeatal angle.
- Use tragal perichondrium for tympanic membrane grafting with the endaural approach and fresh temporalis fascia with the retroauricular approach.
- Do not elevate the tympanic annulus from the sulcus at the "sacred" anterior tympanomeatal angle.

- Be sure to form the new inferoposterior "ledge" of bone at the level of the original tympanic sulcus.
- Place the graft under the malleus handle in subtotal perforations.
- The water test is extremely important for establishing patency of the attic. A negative water test result is an indication for removal of the malleus head and incus, and epitympanectomy, and eventually, posterior tympanotomy may be required.

- Perform an antrotomy whenever eustachian tube function is questionable.
- Carry out an epitympanectomy if the attic is obstructed (water test result negative).

Chapter 3
Ossiculoplasty

General Considerations

1. Basic Situations in Ossiculoplasty

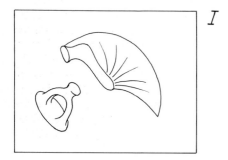

I

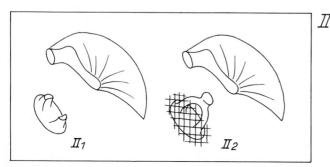

II₁   *II₂*   *II*

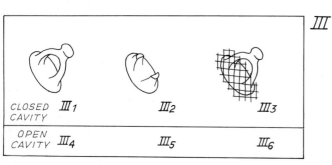

CLOSED *III₁*   *III₂*   *III₃*   *III*
CAVITY

OPEN *III₄*   *III₅*   *III₆*
CAVITY

Fig. 20

The basic situations in reconstruction of the ossicular chain (*ossiculoplasty*) can be divided into three groups according to the expected functional result:

Basic situation I:
Malleus and Stapes
The functional results of ossicular reconstruction in the presence of a mobile intact stapes, the malleus handle, and an intact anterior drum yield, on average, a closure of the air–bone gap to within 10 dB.

Basic situation II:
Malleus and Footplate
The expected average air–bone gap after reconstruction is within 20 dB.

Basic situation III: Stapes only
This ossicular situation can be subdivided in two groups depending upon the type of operative cavity:
a) *closed cavity:* mobile stapes (**III₁**), mobile footplate (**III₂**) and fixed stapes (**III₃**).
b) *open cavity:* mobile stapes (**III₄**), mobile footplate (**III₅**) and fixed stapes (**III₆**). The expected air–bone gap after reconstruction averages 30 dB for both groups.

Specific Surgical Techniques

1. Basic Situation I: Malleus and Stapes, Incus Missing

Only the ossicular reconstruction for the mobile stapes in a closed cavity is considered here. The fixed stapes is handled as for basic situation II$_2$. The open cavities are managed similarly to the closed.

a) Incus Interposition

Surgical Technique

Incus interposition is the preferred type of reconstruction in basic situation I and consists of placing a reshaped incus between the stapes head and malleus handle. An autologous, or rarely, allograft incus is used. The allograft incus is placed in 4% Formalin for 4 weeks and then stored in a mercury compound solution (Cialit 1:500). As an alternative, an incus made from biocompatible materials such as polymaleinate glass Ionomer, (Ionos, Medizinische Produkte, GmbH, Seefeld, Germany) or Hydroxyapatite (Richards, Memphis, Tenn., USA) may also be used. The operation is carried out in one stage, except when the anterior half of the tympanic membrane is absent. A large anterior perforation destabilizes the malleus handle.

The incus interposition is performed similarly in open and closed cavities.

Fig. 21

Principle of incus interposition

A,B: Preservation or removal of the malleus head does not influence the final functional result in a closed cavity.

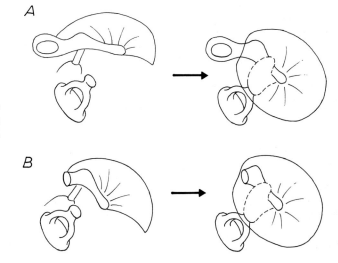

A

B

OPEN CAVITY
(BASIC SITUATION I)

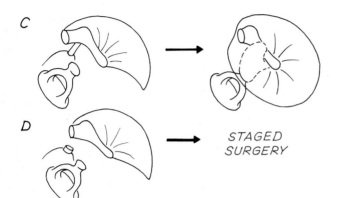

C

D

→ STAGED
SURGERY

Fig. **21** (cont.)

Principle of incus interposition (cont.)

C: In open cavity, preservation of the tensor tympani tendon is essential for a good functional result.

D: The absence of the tensor tympani tendon compromises the final hearing result because of anterior migration of the malleus handle. Therefore, in an open cavity, staged surgery is preferred if the tensor tympani tendon is missing or cut.

Surgical Highlights

- Local anesthesia
- Endaural approach
- Preservation of chorda tympani
- Modification of auto- or allograft incus (notch for the stapes in the short process, notch for the malleus on the articular surface)
- Interposition of modified incus
- Stabilization of the interposed incus with the chorda tympani

Surgical Steps

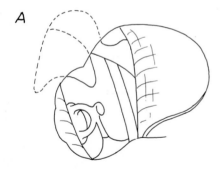

A

Fig. **22 A**

Missing long process of the incus

1.5 mm, 45° HOOK

B

Fig. **22 B**

Removal of the incus

Note rotation of the incus for extraction.

Fig. 22 C

Size and inclination of modified incus

The length of the universal raspatory is 2.5 mm and usually corresponds to the distance between the stapes head and malleus handle. The position of the microraspatory is very useful in assessing the necessary gap to bridge the defect between both ossicles.

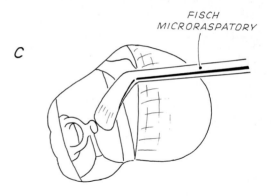

C

FISCH MICRORASPATORY

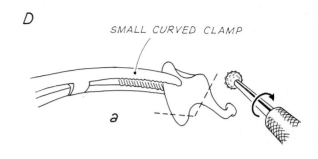

D

SMALL CURVED CLAMP

a

Fig. 22 D

Shaping the incus

a: A small curved clamp holds the incus body so that no change of its position is necessary while drilling. A diamond burr is used to remove the long process of the incus and the posterior part of the incus body.

b: The articular surface of the incus is carved with a drill to accomodate the malleus handle. A notch for the stapes head is drilled in the incus body using a 0.6 mm and an 0.8 mm diamond burr.

d: The correct size and inclination of the interposed incus are determined with the universal microdissector.

e: The interposed incus should fit tightly between the stapes head and proximal malleus handle.

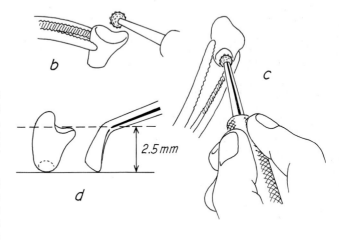

b

c

d

2.5 mm

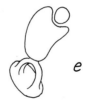

e

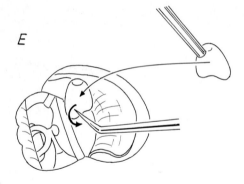

E

Fig. **22 E**

Introduction of the modified incus

The modified incus is picked up with the largest microsuction tube and placed in contact with the malleus handle caudal to the preserved chorda tympani.

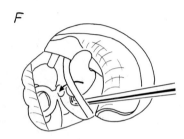

F

Fig. **22 F**

Interposition of modified incus

The modified incus is lateralized and rotated over the stapes head with a 1.5-mm, 45° hook.

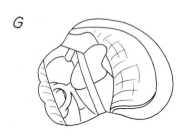

G

Fig. **22 G**

Final position of the interposed incus

The incus is firmly attached to the stapes head and proximal malleus handle (just below the lateral process). The chorda tympani runs cranial to the interposed incus and prevents contact between the incus and the surrounding bone (prevention of fixation).

Fig. **22 H**

Variable inclination of the interposed incus

The distance between the malleus handle and stapes head can vary greatly. Appropriate shaping of the incus is necessary for the stability of the interposed ossicle. Note that the articulation to the malleus is shaped in such a way that the incus body is higher than the malleus handle. This gives better stability to the interposed incus and also affords better contact with the undersurface of the drum.

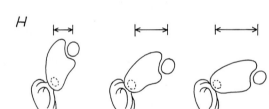

H

a   b   c

Fig. **22 I**

Surgical site after repositioning the tympanomeatal flap

The incus lies just distal to the lateral process of the malleus. The proximal position of the interposed incus along the malleus handle increases the stability of the reconstruction because the maximal movements of the malleus handle when swallowing, sneezing, or blowing the nose occur at the umbo.

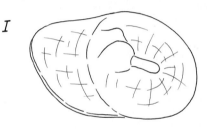

Alternative Technique (Ionomer Ossicle)

Fig. **22 J**

Size and shape of Ionomer incus

A diamond burr is used to sculpt the (5-mm) Ionomer ossicle to the shape of the autologous incus (see Fig. 22 D). The universal microdissector is helpful in determining the size and angulation because its curved tip approximates the average distance between the malleus and stapes (2.5 mm).

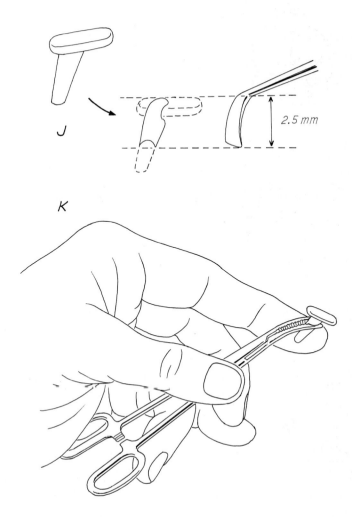

Fig. **22 K**

Stabilization for shaping of the Ionomer ossicle

The shaft of the Ionomer ossicle is fragile and requires careful grasping with the clamp. A specially modified small clamp (Fig. 22 L) is used. The ossicle is stabilized against the index finger and the clamp between the thumb, palm and ring finger. The clamp should not be latched to avoid shattering of the ossicle.

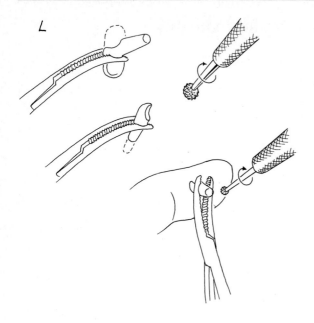

L

Fig. **22 L**

Stabilization for shaping of the Ionomer ossicle (cont.)

The head and shaft are also grasped with the clamp to afford stabilization for further sculpturing.

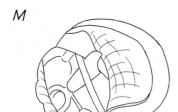

M

Fig. **22 M**

The final position of the Ionomer incus

The Ionomer incus should rest securely between the malleus and stapes as described in Fig. **22 G.**

2. Basic Situation II: Footplate and Malleus

The ossicular reconstructions for the mobile footplate (II$_1$) and fixed footplate (II$_2$) (see Fig. 20) are discussed only for *closed* cavities because the *open* cavities are managed in a similar fashion.

2.1 Basic Situation II$_1$: Mobile Footplate and Malleus, Closed Cavity

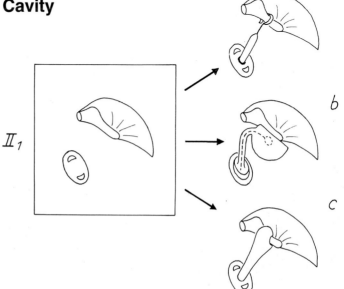

Fig. 23

Alternatives for ossiculo-plasty in basic situation II$_1$.

The alternative techniques for ossiculoplasty in basic situation II$_1$ are:

a Incus replacement with stapedotomy (IRS)
b Spandrel II
c Autograft or biocompatible ossicle

a) Incus Replacement with Stapedotomy (IRS)

Surgical Technique

The operation is performed in one stage if the tympanic membrane is intact. A perforated tympanic membrane requires second-stage surgery. The patients selected for IRS should not demonstrate signs of tubal dysfunction for 6-12 months before surgery. The same 0.4 × 6 mm Teflon Platinum Piston (TPP) (Xomed-Treace [RE No 11-56234]) is used in this procedure as for stapedotomy. A longer 0.4 × 9 mm TPP (Xomed-Treace [RE No 11-56238]) may be necessary in anomalous ears.

Surgical Highlights

- Local anesthesia (as for stapedotomy)
- Endaural approach
- Tympanomeatal flap elevated from the superior half of the handle and lateral process of the malleus
- Manual perforation of mobile footplate
- 0.4-mm TPP attached to superior half of malleus handle and placed in the vestibule
- Sealing of stapedotomy opening with connective tissue, venous blood, and fibrin glue
- Wound closure, packing, and postoperative care as for stapedotomy

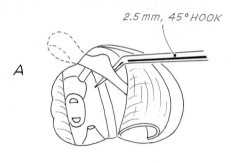

2.5 mm, 45° HOOK

A

Surgical Steps

Fig. 24 A

Exposure of malleus handle

A tympanomeatal flap similar to that used in stapedotomy (see Figs. 107 D–G, p. 216) is elevated exposing the lateral process and the superior half of the malleus handle. This wide exposure eliminates the need for creating a tunnel between the malleus handle and drum for introducing and crimping the prosthesis.

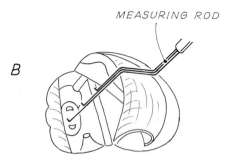

MEASURING ROD

B

Fig. 24 B

Determination of prosthesis length

The stapedotomy measuring rod may be bent to allow accurate placement against the malleus.

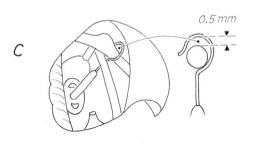

0.5 mm

C

Fig. 24 C

Prosthesis positioned over footplate

A 0.4-mm TPP is trimmed on the stapedotomy cutting block (see Fig. 110 B, p. 220) and introduced in the middle ear with a large alligator forceps (see Figs. 112 A, B, p. 222). The TPP is positioned between the malleus handle and stapes footplate remaining below the preserved chorda tympani. If the length of the prosthesis is correct, its loop lies 0.5 mm higher than the malleus handle allowing for adequate protrusion into the vestibule. If the prosthesis is too long, it is removed for further trimming. A too short prosthesis has to be replaced by a new one. The loop may need to be enlarged to fit the malleus as shown in Fig. 123 I, p. 239.

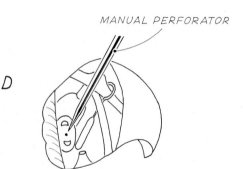

MANUAL PERFORATOR

D

Fig. 24 D

Perforation of mobile footplate

The TPP is moved away from the footplate leaving its loop attached to the malleus. The center of the mobile footplate is opened with manual perforators (see stapedotomy, Figs. 111 A, B, C, p. 221). The diameter of the opening should be slightly larger than 0.4 mm. Manual perforators are preferred to the electric microdrill because they allow better control of the pressure exerted on the mobile footplate during perforation.

Fig. 24 E

Completed stapedotomy

The final opening is visible in the center of the footplate.

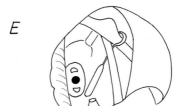

Fig. 24 F

Crimping of the prosthesis to the malleus handle

The TPP is introduced for 0.5 mm into the vestibule.
A fine, straight alligator forceps is used to crimp the prosthesis loop to the malleus handle. The loop should be firmly attached to the full circumference of the malleus handle so that no free movement is possible. The platinum ribbon of the loop conforms better to the shape of the malleus than a stainless steel wire.

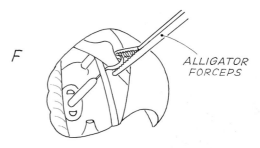

ALLIGATOR FORCEPS

Fig. 24 G

Sealing the stapedotomy

Three connective tissue pledgets obtained from the endaural incision (see Figs. 115 A, B, p. 226) are placed around the stapedotomy opening. Venous blood obtained from the cubital vein of the patient is applied over the oval window. A few drops of fibrin glue are used to reinforce the sealing.

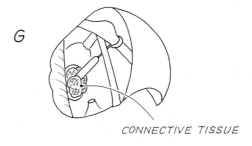

CONNECTIVE TISSUE

Fig. 24 H

Correct position of IRS prosthesis

The TPP loop should be attached adjacent to the lateral process (correct) rather than toward the umbo (incorrect). The correct attachment of the prosthesis to the malleus avoids excessive movements of the piston into the vestibule. The movements of the tip of the malleus handle when sneezing or blowing the nose can reach as much as 1 mm. If correctly placed, the TPP has no adverse effects on the inner ear even after retraction of the drum.

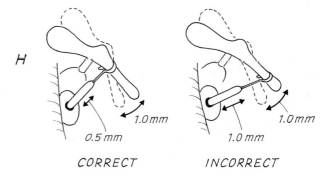

CORRECT   INCORRECT

b) Spandrel II

Surgical Technique

The Spandrel II is used as a one-stage operation only if the tympanic membrane is intact or if at least its anterior half is present.

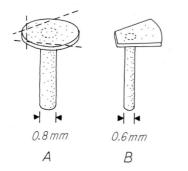

0.8 mm   0.6 mm

A   B

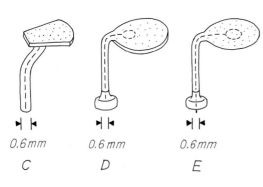

0.6 mm   0.6 mm   0.6 mm

C   D   E

Surgical Highlights

- Local anesthesia
- Tympanomeatal flap as for stapedotomy
- Removal of air from the Spandrel's polycel casing
- Assembly of the Spandrel shaft and shoe
- Transportation of the Spandrel with microsuction tube
- Adaptation of the Spandrel's shoe with spike on the center of the footplate
- Rotation of the Spandrel head under the center of the drum
- Closure and packing as for stapedotomy

Fig. 25

Origin of Spandrel II

A: The Spandrel prosthesis has evolved from Shea's TORP.

B: First the diameter of the shaft was reduced to 0.6 mm and the head of the prosthesis cut in an L shape. The smaller shaft proved to be too soft, and therefore, a stainless steel wire was introduced in the shaft to increase its stability.

C: This change permitted modification of the shape of the shaft according to needs.

D: The head of the TORP was then made round and thinner. A wire platform was introduced in the head for better sound transmission (Spandrel I). A shoe was also developed for better stabilization of the prosthesis over the footplate. The name *Spandrel* originated from the similarity of its shape with that of the triangular space situated beneath the string of a stair that is also called "spandrel."

E: Since 1985 further modifications have led to the Spandrel II. The metal platform was moved to the center of the head. The edge of the head has been made as thin as possible to avoid lesion of the drum by sharp angles. The wire of the shaft was made to protrude a fraction of a millimeter beyond the shoe to serve as an anchoring spike. The sound–collecting and sound–conducting behavior of the Spandrel II has been analyzed by Williams and Lesser (Clin. Otolaryng. 17: 261-270, 1992) using the finite element method. The analysis has examined the mode shapes, displacements, and natural frequencies of the prosthesis for a variety of material properties and geometries. The result indicates that the Spandrel II has better vibration behavior than other available prostheses made of a more rigid material such as ceravital, frialite, hydroxyapatite, and carbon. The advantages of Spandrel II (Xomed–Treace, RE No.: 11-56295) are the ability to keep the shoe firmly in position at the oval window while rotating the head along the undersurface of the drum and the compliance of its head in response to movements of the tympanic membrane. This eliminates the need for covering the prosthesis head with cartilage for protection.

Surgical Steps

Assembly of Spandrel II

Fig. 26 A

The Spandrel II prosthesis

The Spandrel II (Xomed–Treace No.11–56295) consists of two parts: 1) the head with shaft and 2) the shoe. Sound transmission is through the metal platform in the head and the wire core in the shaft. The wire core is made with machined stainless steel wire, 0.12 mm in diameter. The polycel casing (highly refined polyethylene) that forms the head and the shaft stabilizes the sound-transmitting wire core. The shoe of the prosthesis is perforated to allow introduction of the wire core. The hole in the shoe stops 0.2 mm from its base. Advancing the wire core through the last 0.2 mm gives sufficient friction to stabilize the shoe.

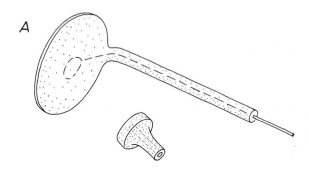

Fig. 26 B

Removal of air from the Spandrel casing

The shaft and shoe of the Spandrel are placed in a syringe containing Ringer's solution and an antibiotic solution (penicillin or tetracycline).

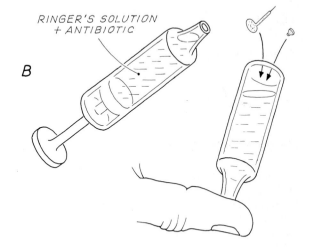

RINGER'S SOLUTION + ANTIBIOTIC

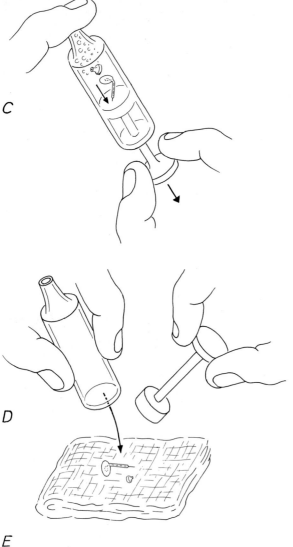

C

Fig. **26 C**

Removal of air from the Spandrel casing (cont.)

The upper end of the syringe is closed with a finger, and the piston of the syringe is pulled back, creating a negative pressure, which removes the air from the pores of the polycel. The deaerated Spandrel sinks according to gravity when the piston of the syringe is released.

Fig. **26 D**

Recovering the Spandrel

The piston of the syringe is removed. The two parts of the prosthesis are emptied onto a wet surgical towel.

D

E

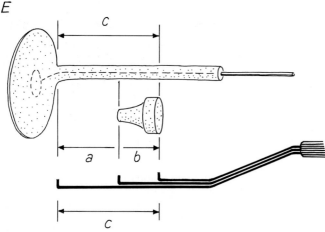

Fig. **26 E**

Determination of Spandrel length

The total length (**c**) of the Spandrel is given by adding the length at the shaft (**a**) and of the shoe (**b**). Before assembly, the polycel casing has to be trimmed to the length a = c−b. The figure shows how the Spandrel and the shoe are aligned for proper length determination. For determination of the total length of the Spandrel see also Fig. 27 A.

Fig. 26 F

Trimming the Spandrel casing

The polycel casing is grasped with a fine dressing forceps proximal to the predetermined length **a** (see Fig. 26 E) and cut with a No. 11 blade.

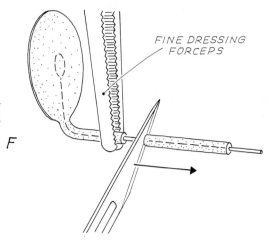

F

FINE DRESSING FORCEPS

G

Fig. 26 G

Perforation of the Spandrel shoe

A 0.3-mm manual perforator (see stapedotomy) is used to make a hole in the shoe. This step is superfluous if a Spandrel II (No. 11-56295) is used because its shoe is perforated with exception of the last 0.2 mm by the manufacturer (see Fig. 26 A).

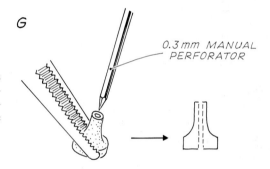

0.3 mm MANUAL PERFORATOR

H

Fig. 26 H

Cutting the Spandrel's wire core

The wire core is cut with wire scissors so that it is 0.5 mm longer than the base of the shoe (**b** + 0.5mm).

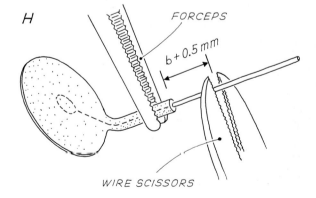

FORCEPS

$b + 0.5$ mm

WIRE SCISSORS

I

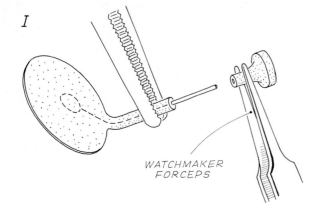

WATCHMAKER
FORCEPS

Fig. 26 I

Assembly of the Spandrel

The shoe is grasped with watchmaker forceps and introduced over the wire core.

J

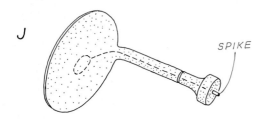

SPIKE

Fig. 26 J

The assembled Spandrel

The Spandrel shoe is in position. The wire core protrudes 0.5 mm from the shoe (spike).

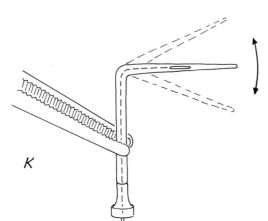

K

Fig. 26 K

Angulation of the Spandrel head

The position of the Spandrel head is adjusted to the position of the tympanic membrane.

Introduction of Spandrel II

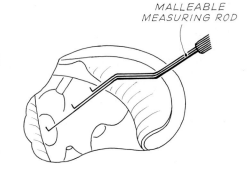

MALLEABLE
MEASURING ROD

A

Fig. 27 A

Determination of the Spandrel's length

The distance between the drum and stapes foot-plate is determined with the malleable measuring rod (see stapedotomy, Fig. 110 A, p. 220). The prosthesis is assembled as shown in Figs. 26 A–K.

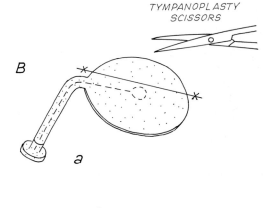

TYMPANOPLASTY
SCISSORS

B

a

Fig. 27 B

Shaping of the Spandrel's head

In basic situation II₁, the anterior half of the Spandrel head is cut away with tympanoplasty scissors (**a**) to bring the prosthesis in contact with the malleus handle (**b**).

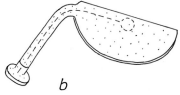

b

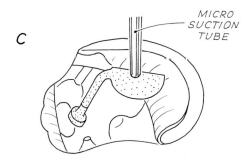

MICRO
SUCTION
TUBE

C

Fig. 27 C

Transportation of the Spandrel

The assembled Spandrel is stored on a wet dressing towel. For transportation, the head of the prosthesis is picked up with a large microsuction tube.

D

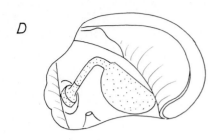

Fig. 27 D

Positioning of Spandrel on the footplate

The shoe of the Spandrel is placed with its spike on the center of the mobile footplate. The curved shape of the shaft gives an excellent view of the oval window during this step of the procedure.

E

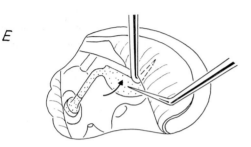

Fig. 27 E

Rotation of the Spandrel head under the center of the drum

The tympanic membrane is elevated with 0.5-mm, 90° hook (left hand). The prosthesis head is rotated against the malleus handle using a 2.5-mm, 45° hook (right hand).

F

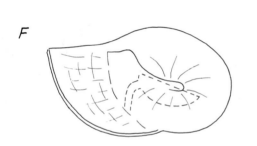

Fig. 27 F

Repositioning of tympanomeatal flap

The tympanomeatal flap is reflected into its original position. The Spandrel head (*broken line*) is in contact with the malleus handle.

G

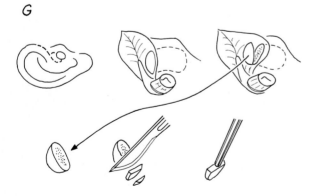

Fig. 27 G

Stabilization of the Spandrel shoe: harvesting of tragal cartilage

Additional stabilization is required in a wide oval window niche. Cartilage is obtained from the cranial edge of the tragus, taking advantage of the initial endaural incision. A piece of tragal cartilage is cut into smaller fragments, which are picked up with a large microsuction tube.

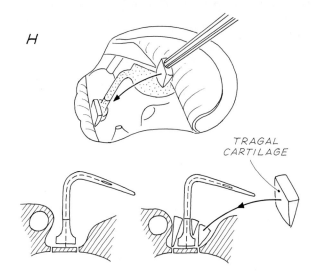

Fig. **27 H**

Stabilization of the Spandrel foot: tragal cartilage in the oval window niche

The tympanomeatal flap is elevated again. A few pieces of tragal cartilage are placed in the oval window niche to stabilize the Spandrel shoe.

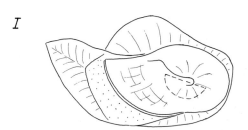

Fig. **27 I**

Repositioning of tympanomeatal flap

The tympanomeatal flap is back in its original position. The broken line shows the Spandrel head in contact with the malleus handle.

c) Use of Autograft Ossicles

Surgical Technique

The first and last steps are performed as in stapedotomy (see Figs. **107 A-G, 116 A, B,** pp. 215–217 and 226–227).

Surgical Highlights

- Local anesthesia
- Tympanomeatal flap as for stapedotomy
- Shaping of ossicle with diamond burr
- Fixation of ossicle on stapes footplate with connective tissue and fibrin glue
- Fixation of ossicle on malleus handle with carved notch

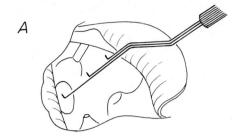

A

Surgical Steps

Fig. 28 A

Determination of the ossicle's length

A malleable measuring rod (see stapedotomy) is used to determine the distance between the footplate and malleus handle.

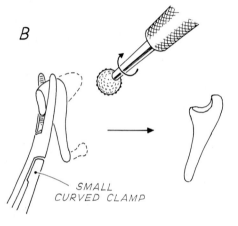

B

SMALL
CURVED CLAMP

Fig. 28 B

Shaping the autograft incus

The ossicle is grasped with a small curved clamp. The lenticular process and the short process are removed with a diamond burr. The articular surface is modified for better contact with the malleus handle.

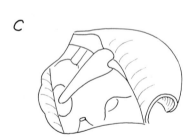

C

Fig. 28 C

Ossicle in place

The modified incus is interposed between the center of the footplate and the upper half of the malleus handle.

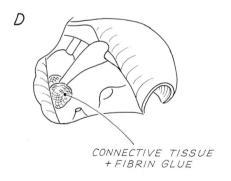

D

CONNECTIVE TISSUE
+ FIBRIN GLUE

Fig. 28 D

Stabilization of the ossicle

The long process of the incus is stabilized on the footplate with connective tissue pledgets and fibrin glue. Tragal cartilage can also be used for this purpose (see Figs. 27 G, H).

LATERALIZATION
n = 15

50 %

FISH. 29

Causes of failure of the ossicular chain with autograft incus after reconstruction.

The failure in 30 cases of one-stage ossicular chain reconstruction with autograft ossicles (incus or malleus) was due to:

1. lateralization (50% of the cases)
2. bony fixation (20% of the cases)
3. atrophy (13.3% of the cases)
4. displacement (13.3% of the cases)
5. perforation of the stapes footplate with perilymphatic fistula (3.3% of the cases)

FIXATION
n = 6

20 %

ATROPHY
n = 4

13.3 %

DISPLACEMENT
n = 4

13.3 %

FISTULA
n = 1

3.3 %

Biocompatible ossicles, particularly Ionomer ossicles are increasingly used when autograft ossicles are not available.

2.2 Basic Situation II₂: Fixed Footplate and Malleus, Closed Cavity

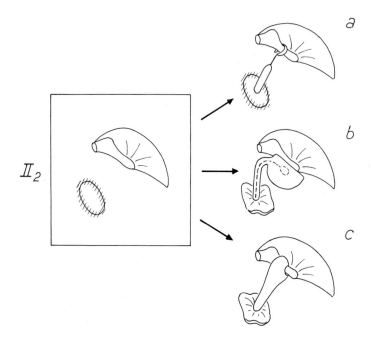

Fig. 30

Alternative methods for ossiculoplasty in basic situation II₂

The alternatives for ossiculoplasty in the presence of a fixed stapes and malleus handles are
a: Incus replacement with stapedotomy (IRS)
b: Spandrel and stapedectomy
c: Autograft or biocompatible ossicle and stapedectomy

a) Incus Replacement with Stapedotomy (IRS)

The technique of incus replacement with stapedotomy (IRS) for a fixed footplate and malleus handle is similar to that described for the mobile footplate in basic situation II₁ (see Figs. **24A–H**). IRS is the first-choice ossiculoplasty for basic situation II₂. Candidates for this operation should not have evidence of tubal dysfunction in the previous 6–12 months and should present with an intact drum.

b) Spandrel II and Stapedectomy

This is the second-choice ossiculoplasty in basic situation II₂. It is used when the position of malleus handle is too anterior for IRS

or if the malleus handle is too atrophic for fixation of a TPP.

Surgical Technique

The first and last steps of surgery are done as for stapedectomy (see Figs. **107A–G** and **116A, B**, pp. 215–17 and 226–7).

Surgical Highlights

- Local anesthesia
- Endaural approach
- Total stapedectomy
- Covering of the oval window with pressed tragal perichondrium
- Use of Spandrel with spike but without shoe

Surgical Steps

Fig. 31 A

Total stapedectomy

The stapes footplate is first fractured in the midline and then removed in two or more fragments, using a 0.2-mm footplate elevator (see stapedectomy, Figs. 118 G, H, p. 229).

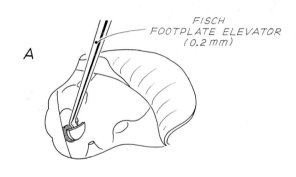

A

FISCH
FOOTPLATE ELEVATOR
(0.2 mm)

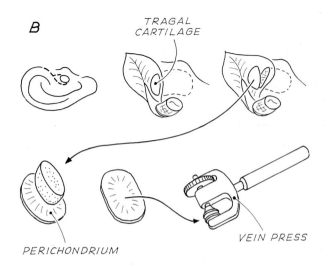

B

TRAGAL
CARTILAGE

PERICHONDRIUM

VEIN PRESS

Fig. 31 B

Harvesting and preparation of the tragal perichondrium

Tragal perichondrium is used to cover the opened oval window. The perichondrium is obtained from the cranial end of the tragal cartilage, which has been exposed by the endaural incision. A Shea vein press is used to reduce the thickness of the perichondrium.

Fig. 31 C

Covering of the oval window with pressed perichondrium

The perichondrium is picked up and transported with a 1.5-mm, 45° hook.

C

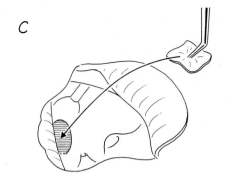

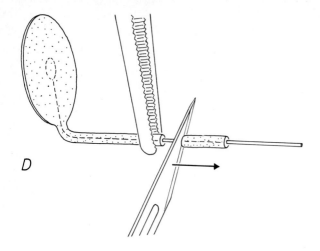

D

Fig. 31 D

Trimming the Spandrel's polycel casing

No shoe is used in this situation. The Spandrel casing is cut to the desired length using a No. 11 blade.

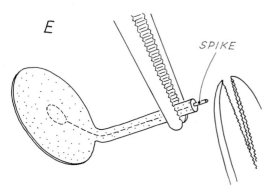

E

SPIKE

Fig. 31 E

Cutting the wire core

The wire core is cut with wire scissors leaving a 0.5-mm spike for fixation on the perichondrial graft covering the oval window.

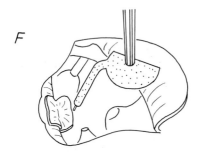

F

Fig. 31 F

Reduction of the Spandrel's head and transportation into the middle ear

The anterior third of the Spandrel's head is removed to allow alignment of the prosthesis close to the malleus handle. The Spandrel is introduced into the middle ear by means of a large microsuction tube.

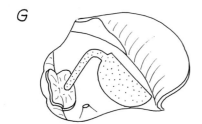

G

Fig. 31 G

Spandrel on oval window

The Spandrel's shaft with spike rests in the middle of the perichondrium covering the oval window.

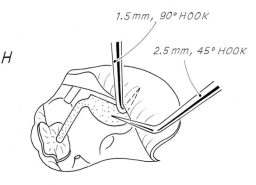

Fig. 31 H

Rotation of the Spandrel's head

The drum is raised with a 1.5-mm, 90° hook (left hand) and the head of the Spandrel is rotated against the malleus handle with a 2.5-mm, 45° hook (right hand).

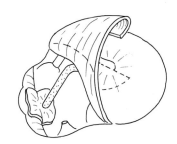

Fig. 31 I

Final position of Spandrel

The Spandrel is in position between the oval window and the malleus handle. The tympanomeatal flap is ready for replacement.

c) Autograft or Biocompatible Ossicle and Stapedectomy

The indications are the same as those for Spandrel II. The Spandrel is preferred because of its superior functional results. An ossicle is used in cases with marginal tubal function.

Surgical Technique

The first and last steps of the procedure are done as for stapedotomy (see Figs. **107A–G** and **116A**, **B**, pp. 215–217 and 226–227).

Surgical Highlights

- Local anesthesia
- Total stapedectomy
- Modified autograft incus interposed between the oval window and malleus handle

A

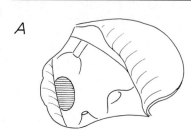

Surgical Steps

Fig. **32 A**

Total stapedectomy

(see also Fig. 31 A).

B

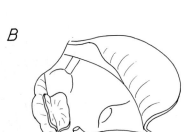

Fig. **32 B**

Covering of the oval window with pressed tra-gal perichondrium

(see also Figs. 31 B–C).

C

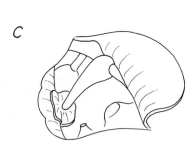

Fig. **32 C**

Modified autograft incus interposed between oval window and malleus handle

(see also Figs. 28 A–D).

3. Basic Situation III: Stapes Only

The stapes only situation (basic situation III) is discussed separately for

a) *closed cavity*, and
b) *open cavity*.

4. Basic Situation III₁, III₂, III₃: Stapes Only in Closed Cavity

Depending on the integrity and mobility of the stapes, the ossiculoplasty in a *stapes only, closed cavity* situation may be divided into the following subtypes:

III₁ = mobile stapes
III₂ = mobile footplate
III₃ = fixed footplate

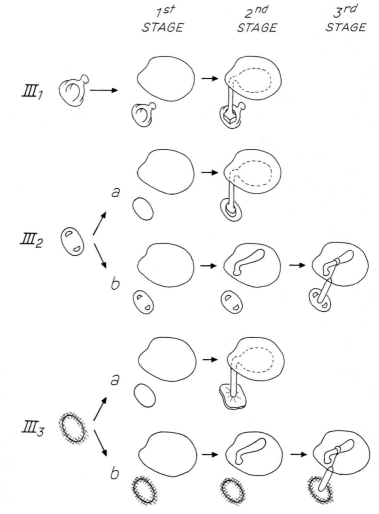

Fig. 33

Alternative techniques of ossiculoplasty in stapes only and closed cavity

The alternative techniques of ossiculoplasty in this situation are:

– III₁ (mobile stapes): Spandrel II

– III₂ (mobile footplate): (*a*) Spandrel II or (*b*) neomalleus with incus replacement and stapedotomy (NMIRS)

– III₃ (fixed stapes): (*a*) Spandrel II with stapedectomy or (*b*) neomalleus with incus replacement and stapedotomy (NMIRS)

4.1 Basic Situation III₁: Mobile Stapes, Closed Cavity

In this situation, the first-choice ossiculoplasty is the use of Spandrel II. Other alternatives are: (a) the interposition of an autograft or biocompatible ossicle between the stapes head and drum and (b) the neomalleus with incus interposition and stapedotomy (NMIRS).

a) Spandrel II

Surgical Technique

The operation is performed in one stage if the tympanic membrane is intact. The first and last steps are similar to those for stapedotomy (see Figs. **107 A–G,** pp. 215–217, and **116 A –B,** pp. 226–227).

Surgical Highlights

- Local anesthesia
- Spandrel (with shoe and spike) interposed between mobile stapes and tympanic membrane

Surgical Steps

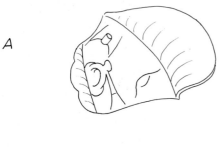

A

Fig. 34 A

Exposure of oval window niche

The tympanomeatal flap is raised, exposing the mobile stapes. The cavity is closed (basic situation III₁).

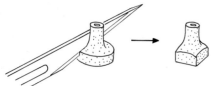

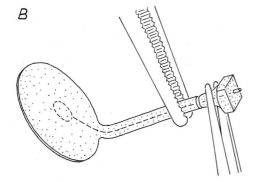

B

Fig. 34 B

Trimming of the Spandrel shoe

The shaft and wire core of the Spandrel are cut as shown in Figs. 26 E, F, G, and H. The size of the Spandrel shoe is reduced with a No. 11 blade to allow it to fit between the stapes crura. The Spandrel is assembled, leaving 0.5 mm of the wire core (spike) protruding from the shoe (see also Fig. 26 J).

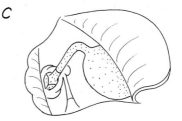

Fig. 34 C

Spandrel on footplate

The Spandrel shoe fits between the crura. The stapes arch helps stabilize the prosthesis shaft.

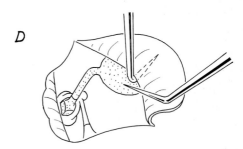

Fig. 34 D

Rotation of the Spandrel's head under the drum

The tympanic membrane is raised with a 1.5-mm, 90° hook (left hand). The head of the Spandrel is rotated under the center of the drum.

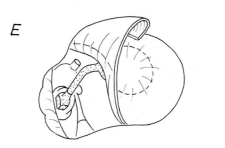

Fig. 34 E

Spandrel in position

The final position of the Spandrel is reached when the prosthesis fits, under slight tension, between the footplate of the stapes and the center of the drum.

b) Autograft or Biocompatible Ossicle

This technique is used when eustachian tube function is marginal because ossicles can accept severe retraction of the drum without extrusion. The functional results are not as good as those of Spandrel II because the reconstruction is not as stable (see results, p. 108).

Surgical Technique

The first and last steps of the procedure are done as for stapedotomy (see Figs. **107A–G** and **116A**, **B**, pp. 215–217 and 226–227).

Surgical Highlights

- Local anesthesia
- Modification of autograft incus or biocompatible ossicle
- Interposition of ossicle between the stapes head and drum

Surgical Steps

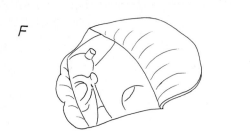

F

Fig. 34 F

Exposure of oval window niche

Surgical site showing the mobile stapes in a closed cavity (second stage).

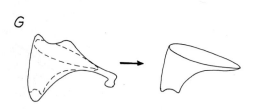

G

Fig. 34 G

Modification of autograft incus

The patient's incus, which was preserved from the first stage, is soaked in Ringer's solution. The notch for the stapes head is made on the short process of the incus. The articular surface and the long process are flattened for proper contact with the drum.

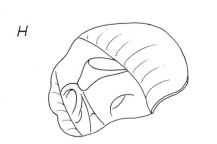

H

Fig. 34 H

Modified incus in place

The ossicular columella is in position between the stapes head and drum. The tympanomeatal flap was raised just enough for visualization while still maintaining sufficient tension for stabilization of the interposed ossicle.

Alternative Technique

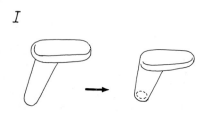

I

Fig. 34 I

Modification of glass Ionomer ossicle (see instrumentation)

A 5-mm Ionos ossicle is modified with a diamond burr (see Figs. 22 J , K, L, M) for interposition between the stapes head and drum.

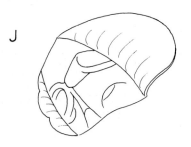

J

Fig. 34 J

Ionos ossicle in position

The modified Ionos ossicle is kept in position by the tension of the drum.

4.2 Basic Situation III₂: Mobile Footplate, Closed Cavity

a) Spandrel II

Surgical Technique

The Spandrel II is the first choice because it carries a very low risk of inner ear damage. The neomalleus with incus replacement and stapedotomy (NMIRS) gives better functional results but has a higher potential risk of sensorineural hearing loss.

The Spandrel II is most often used as a second-stage procedure. One-stage surgery is possible in the presence of an intact tympanic membrane. The first and last steps of surgery are performed with local anesthesia as for stapedotomy (see Figs. **107 A–G** and **116A, B**, pp. 215–217 and 226–227).

Surgical Highlights

- Spandrel II with shoe and spike interposed between the mobile footplate and drum

Surgical Steps

For the preparation, transportation, and introduction of the Spandrel, see Figs. **27A–D**.

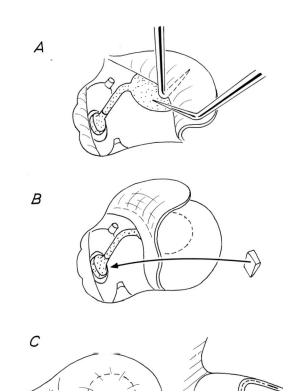

Fig. **35 A**   A

Rotation of the Spandrel's head under drum

The Spandrel shoe with spike is placed on the mobile footplate. The head of the Spandrel is rotated under the center of the drum using two hooks.

Fig. **35 B**   B

Stabilization of the Spandrel shoe

Pieces of cartilage are used to stabilize the Spandrel shoe in the oval window niche (see also Figs. 27 G–H).

Fig. **35 C**   C

Final position of the Spandrel

The prosthesis head lies under the center of the drum. The angulation of the head corresponds to the position of the drum. The prosthesis shoe is stabilized by pieces of tragal cartilage in the oval window.

b) Neomalleus and Incus Replacement with Stapedotomy (NMIRS)

Surgical Technique

The neomalleus ossiculoplasty is usually performed in two stages. In the *first stage*, the new malleus is incorporated in the tragal perichondrium and placed as an underlay graft over the oval window. In the *second stage*, the incus replacement with stapedotomy (IRS) is performed. A single-stage operation is possible if the tympanic membrane is thick enough to permit creation of a pouch for the introduction and fixation of the neomalleus. Patient selection is critical. There should be no signs of tubal dysfunction for 6–12 months prior to reconstruction.

Surgical Highlights

First Stage (Perichondrium and Neomalleus)

- Local anesthesia
- Modified autograft or biocompatible incus attached to tragal perichondrium
- Underlay graft of tragal perichondrium with neomalleus
- Posterosuperior and anteroinferior fixation of perichondrial graft between tympanic sulcus and annulus

Second Stage (Incus Replacement with Stapedotomy)

- Local anesthesia
- Stapedotomy with 0.4-mm TPP attached to neomalleus
- Sealing of stapedotomy opening with connective tissue, venous blood, and fibrin glue

Surgical Steps

First Stage (Perichondrium and Neomalleus)

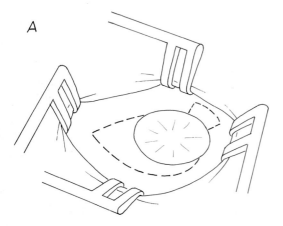

A

Fig. 36 A

Incision for tympanomeatal flaps

The external canal is enlarged with endaural retractors. The endaural incision is usually unnecessary because the patient has had an adequate canalplasty at the first procedure. The posterosuperior tympanomeatal flap is carried out similar to stapedotomy. The anteroinferior flap is rectangular and limited to the area between 4 o'clock and 5 o'clock (right side).

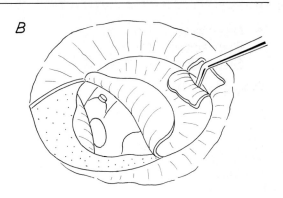

B

Fig. 36 B

Elevation of tympanomeatal flaps

Care is taken to elevate the tympanic annulus from the bony sulcus in both tympanomeatal flaps.

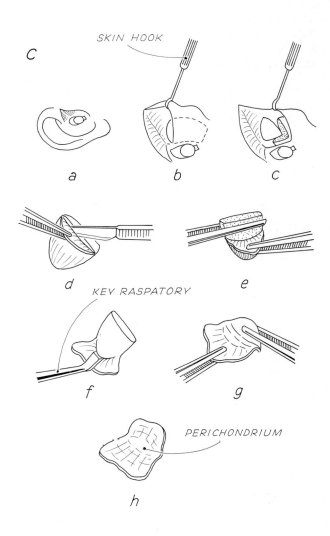

C

Fig. 36 C

Harvesting of tragal perichondrium

a, b: The cranial edge of the tragal cartilage is exposed by the initial endaural incision.

c: A triangular piece of tragal cartilage with perichondrium is excised.

d: The perichondrium is separated from the cartilage using a No. 15 blade.

e: The elevated periostium is grasped with fine dressing forceps and peeled away from the cartilage.

f: The Key raspatory is used to separate the perichondrium around the edge of the cartilage.

g: The thinner perichondrium of the posterior surface of the cartilage is also peeled away with fine dressing forceps.

h: The perichondrium is ready for use.

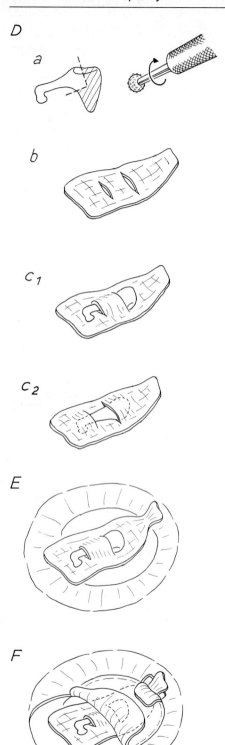

Fig. **36 D**

Modification of incus and incorporation of the neomalleus in tragal perichondrium

a: The short process and the upper portion of the body of the incus are removed with the burr.

b: The perichondrium is placed over a glass board (see also Fig. 14 F), and two incisions are made through it with a No. 11 blade.

c₁: The neomalleus (modified incus) is placed through the perichondrial incisions. The long process lies over the perichondrium.

c₂: The long process of the incus lies under the perichondrium. The advantage is the better stabilization of the neomalleus. The disadvantage is a more rapid resorption.

Fig. **36 E**

Schematic position of neomalleus

Schematic view showing the position of the "neomalleus" over the oval window niche.

Fig. **36 F**

Introduction of perichondrium with neomalleus under the tympanic membrane

The anteroinferior fixation is obtained by pulling the perichondrium through the gap between the tympanic annulus and sulcus by means of a micro-suction tube.

Fig. 36 G

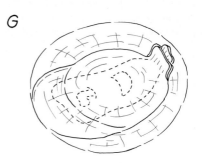

Repositioning of the tympanomeatal flaps

The broken line gives the position of the underlaid perichondrium and neomalleus.

Second Stage
(Incus Replacement and Stapedotomy)

The second stage is performed 3 to 6 months after the first if no signs of tubal dysfunction have appeared.

Fig. 36 H

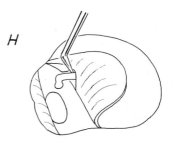

Elevation of the tympanomeatal flap, exposure of the long process of the incus, and preparation of the TPP

The tympanomeatal flap is elevated, and the tip of the long process of the incus is exposed with a 1.5-mm, 45° hook from the soft tissues at the undersurface of the drum. The distance between the footplate and incus is determined with a measuring rod and a 0.4-mm TPP trimmed on a cutting block as described for stapedotomy (see Figs. 110 A, B, C, p. 220). The correct length is verified in situ prior to stapedotomy.

MANUAL
PERFORATOR
(0.3, 0.4, 0.5 mm)

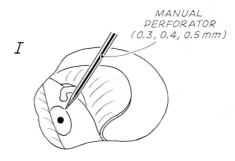

Fig. 36 I

Perforation of mobile footplate

A 0.4-mm stapedotomy is made in the center part of the mobile footplate with manual perforators (see Fig. 111 A, B, C, p. 221).

Fig. 36 J

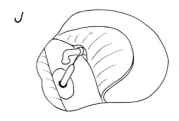

Introduction of a 0.4-mm TPP

The TPP is grasped with the large alligator forceps and introduced into the middle ear. The same forceps are used to crimp the prosthesis loop to the incus. The TPP protrudes 0.5 mm into the vestibule (see stapedotomy Fig. 112 E, p. 223).

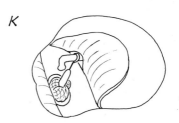

Fig. 36 K

Sealing of stapedotomy

The stapedotomy is sealed with connective tissue pledgets from the endaural incision, venous blood from the cubital vein, and fibrin glue.

One-Stage Neomalleus with Incus Replacement and Stapedotomy (NMIRS)

If the tympanic membrane is sufficiently thick to accomodate the neomalleus, the ossiculoplasty is performed in one stage. A glass Ionomer ossicle can be used in place of the autograft incus. An Ionomer ossicle does not undergo resorption like an autograft incus. For this reason we now favor the use of an Ionomer ossicle even in a two-stage ossiculoplasty.

M

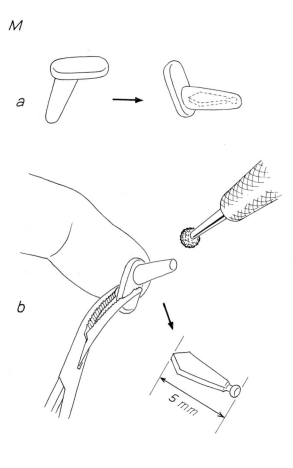

a

b

Fig. 36 M

Shaping of Ionomer "neomalleus"

a: The shaft of a Ionomer ossicle is modified with a diamond burr to the shape of a flat rod with a length of 5 mm. The smaller end of the rod carries a circular indentation to which the prosthesis loop will be crimped.

b: The Ionomer ossicle is easily modified by drilling. However, the material is quite fragile. Therefore, the modified curved clamp used for ossicle fixation should not be completely closed, but kept secured between thumb, palm, and little finger (see Fig. 22 K). The tip of the index finger also helps stabilize the ossicle while drilling.

N

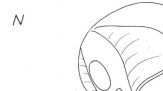

Fig. 36 N

Elevation of tympanomeatal flap

The tympanomeatal flap is elevated as for stapedotomy exposing the mobile footplate.

Fig. 36 O

Formation of a pouch for the neomalleus in the tympanic membrane

For one-stage neomalleus ossiculoplasty, the tympanic membrane should be thick enough to allow formation of a pouch to accomodate and stabilize the neomalleus. The pouch is made in the central tympanic membrane using tympanoplasty microscissors.

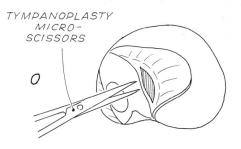

TYMPANOPLASTY
MICRO-
SCISSORS

O

Fig. 36 P

Formation of a pouch for the neomalleus in the tympanic membrane (cont.)

The broken line shows the extent of the pouch created in the tympanic membrane for the neomalleus.

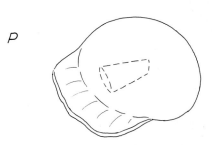

P

Fig. 36 Q

Introduction of Ionomer neomalleus into the tympanic membrane

The Ionomer neomalleus is inserted into the pouch leaving the smaller, rounded end with the notch for the prosthesis protruding over the mobile footplate.

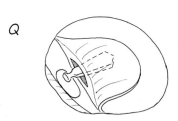

Q

Fig. 36 R

Introduction and fixation of 0.4-mm TPP to the neomalleus

The distance between the stapes footplate and incus has been determined with a measuring rod. A 0.4-mm TPP is trimmed to the desired length on a cutting block (see Figs. 110 B, C, p. 220). The prosthesis is introduced into the middle ear and attached to the notch of the rounded end of the neomalleus with straight alligator forceps. The length of the TPP is such that the TPP protrudes 0.5 mm into the vestibule when the tympanomeatal flap is reflected into its original position.

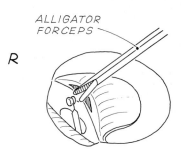

ALLIGATOR
FORCEPS

R

Fig. 36 S

Stapedotomy

After its proper length has been confirmed, the TPP is displaced posteriorly, and a 0.4-mm opening is made in the center of the mobile footplate with manual perforators.

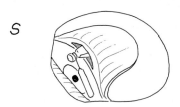

S

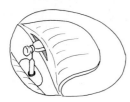

Fig. **36 T**

Introduction of TPP into the vestibule

The TPP is moved over the stapedotomy and introduced for 0.5 mm into the vestibule by lowering the tympanomeatal flap to the level of the tympanic sulcus.

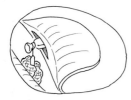

Fig. **36 U**

Sealing of stapedotomy opening

The mucosa surrounding the oval window is scraped with a 0.2-mm footplate elevator. Connective tissue pledgets from the endaural incision, venous blood from the cubital vein of the patient and fibrin glue are used to seal the stapedotomy.

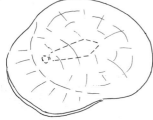

Fig. **36 V**

Final position of neomalleus and TPP

The tympanomeatal flap is replaced. The broken line shows the position of the Ionomer neomalleus (see instrumentation) with attached TPP.

4.3 Basic Situation III₃: Fixed Footplate, Closed Cavity

There are two alternative ossiculoplasties for basic situation III₃ (fixed footplate, closed cavity):

a) Spandrel II and stapedectomy
b) Neomalleus with IRS

the danger of sensorineural hearing loss, which is higher in total stapedectomy than in stapedotomy.

As for all operations requiring opening of the vestibule, this ossiculoplasty is carried out in one stage only in the presence of an intact tympanic membrane to avoid infection. The first and last steps of surgery are the same as for stapedotomy (see Figs. **107 A–G**, pp. 215–217, and **116 A–B**, pp. 226–227).

a) Spandrel II and Stapedectomy

Surgical Technique

This technique is simpler than NMIRS and is carried out in one stage. The disadvantage is the difficult formation of a sufficiently large oval window in an ossified niche and

Surgical Highlights

- Local anesthesia
- Total stapedectomy
- Perichondrium over oval window
- Spandrel with spike but without foot interposed between the oval window and tympanic membrane.

Surgical Steps

Fig. 37 A

Total stapedectomy

The total removal of the footplate is performed as in stapedectomy for otosclerosis (see Figs. 118 G, H, p. 229).

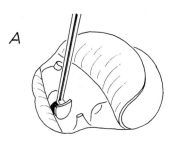

A

Fig. 37 B

Perichondrium covering oval window

A piece of pressed tragal perichondrium (see Figs. 31 B–C, p. 65) is placed over the open oval window.

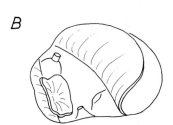

B

Fig. 37 C

Preparation and introduction of Spandrel

The distance between the oval window and tympanic membrane is determined with a measuring rod. The Spandrel shaft and wire core are cut to the desired length. The Spandrel shaft with spike (but without shoe) is placed over the perichondrium at the oval window. The Spandrel head is rotated under the central portion of the tympanic membrane using two hooks.

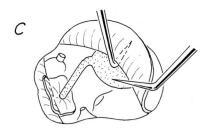

C

Fig. 37 D

Final position of Spandrel

The Spandrel II without foot is firmly in position between the oval window and central portion of the tympanic membrane.

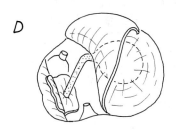

D

b) Neomalleus with Incus Replacement and Stapedotomy (NMIRS)

This ossiculoplasty is carried out as for the mobile footplate (see basic situation III-2, Figs. 36 A–K, pp. 74–77).

The NMIRS ossiculoplasty is the method of choice in basic situation III₃ (fixed footplate, closed cavity). The functional results are better, and the risk is lower than for stapedectomy and Spandrel. The disadvantage is an additional surgical stage.

5. Basic Situation III₄, III₅, and III₆: Stapes Only in Open Cavity

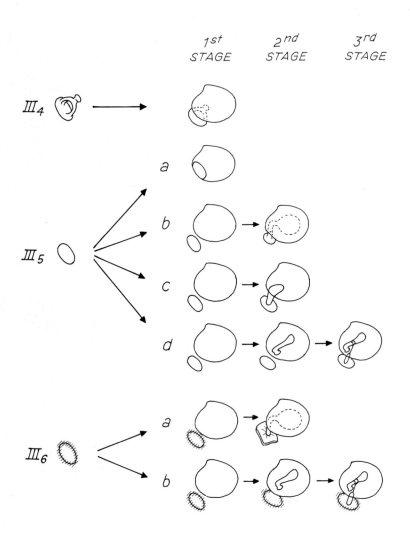

Fig. 38

Alternative ossiculoplasties for basic situations III₄, III₅, and III₆

The alternative techniques of ossiculoplasty for stapes only, open cavity are:

Basic situation III₄ (intact, mobile stapes):
– type III tympanoplasty

Basic situation III₅ (mobile footplate)
a: Type IV tympanoplasty
b: Spandrel II
c: Autograft or biocompatible ossicle
d: NMIRS

Basic situation III₆ (fixed stapes)
a: Spandrel II with Stapedectomy
b: NMIRS

5.1 Basic Situation III₄: Stapes Only, Open Cavity

a) Type III Tympanoplasty with Underlay Grafting of the Tympanic Membrane

Surgical Technique

The type III tympanoplasty is the choice in basic situation III₄. The type III tympanoplasty is a one-stage procedure carried out in conjunction with an open cavity (see open mastoido-epitympanectomy, p. 181).

Type III ossiculoplasty is characterized by impressive, stable long-term results (see results, p. 114).

Surgical Highlights

- General anesthesia
- Preservation of anterior tympanic membrane remnant
- Posterosuperior tympanic sulcus lower than stapes head
- Anterior underlay grafting
- Posterior overlay grafting
- Graft directly over stapes head

Surgical Steps

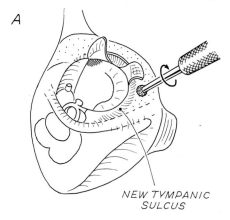

A

NEW TYMPANIC SULCUS

Fig. 39 A

Drilling of a new tympanic sulcus

The remnant tympanic membrane with the attached meatal skin is intact along the "sacred" anterior tympanomeatal angle (see Fig. 12). A ledge of bone (tympanic sulcus) is drilled with a diamond burr along the inferoposterior wall of the tympanic cavity at the level of the stapedial muscle and pyramidal process.

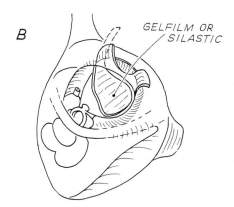

B

GELFILM OR SILASTIC

Fig. 39 B

Sheeting of the middle ear and eustachian tube

Gelfilm or Silastic sheeting is introduced into the epitympanum and into the proximal eustachian tube if the mucosa covering the promontory is defective (see Figs. 49, 50, 51, pp. 99–100, and Figs. 57, 58, p. 107). Gelfilm is used instead of Silastic in the presence of chronically infected middle ear osa.

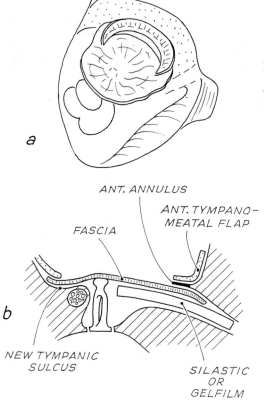

C

a

ANT. ANNULUS

ANT. TYMPANO-
MEATAL FLAP

FASCIA

b

NEW TYMPANIC
SULCUS

SILASTIC
OR
GELFILM

Fig. **39 C**

Anterior underlay and posterior overlay of temporalis fascia

a: The temporalis fascia is placed under the anterior tympanic membrane and over the new posterior tympanic sulcus. The graft also covers the tympanic fallopian canal and the semicircular canal of the tensor tympani muscle. The head of the stapes protrudes above the level of the covering fascia.

b: Cross section showing the position of the fascial graft. The contact with the anterior undersurface of the tympanic membrane is assured by Silastic or Gelfilm sheeting. The new posterior tympanic sulcus is lower than the head of the stapes. The protrusion of the stapes head is essential for good functional results.

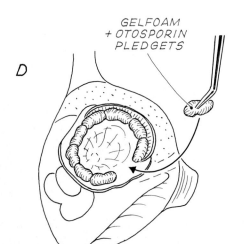

GELFOAM
+ OTOSPORIN
PLEDGETS

D

Fig. **39 D**

Fixation of the graft

The graft is kept in place with Gelfoam pledgets soaked in Otosporin. The anterior tympanomeatal skin is in position.

b) Type III Tympanoplasty with Overlay Grafting of Tympanic Membrane

Surgical Technique

Type III tympanoplasty with overlay grafting is used when the tympanic membrane is absent. The disadvantage of this technique is the possible lateralization of the anterior tympanomeatal angle reducing the possible hearing gain. This is a one-stage procedure. The steps for the open cavity are illustrated for open mastoido-epitympanectomy (p. 182).

Surgical Highlights

- General anesthesia
- Drilling of circumferential ledge of bone
- Graft placed and secured on the new tympanic sulcus
- Stapes head protruding above the level of the overlaid fascia

Surgical Steps

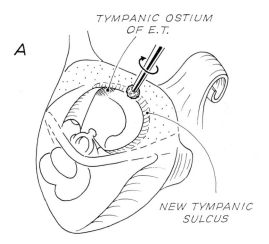

A

TYMPANIC OSTIUM OF E.T.

NEW TYMPANIC SULCUS

Fig. 40 A

Drilling of new tympanic sulcus

In overlay grafting, it is particularly important to drill a well-defined anterior ledge of bone (sulcus) to avoid blunting or lateralization of the anterior tympanomeatal angle.

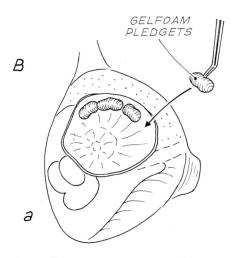

GELFOAM PLEDGETS

B

a

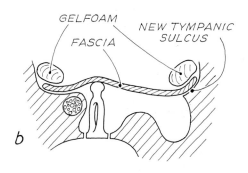

GELFOAM **NEW TYMPANIC SULCUS**
FASCIA

b

Fig. 40 B

Overlay of fascial graft

a: The overlaid fascia is placed on the new tympanic sulcus, on the tympanic fallopian canal, and on the semicanal of the tensor tympani muscle. Fixation on the supporting ledge of bone is obtained with Gelfoam pledgets soaked in Otosporin.

b: Cross section showing the fixation of the overlaid fascia with Gelfoam pledgets soaked in Otosporin. The overlaid fascia extends only a few millimeters beyond the supporting ledge of bone. The stapes head is higher than the new tympanic sulcus and fallopian canal.

5.2 Basic Situation III₅: Mobile Footplate, Open Cavity

a) Type IV Tympanoplasty

Surgical Technique

As for type III tympanoplasty, the fascial graft is underlaid or overlaid depending on the presence or absence of the tympanic membrane. Only type IV tympanoplasty with underlay technique is presented. For type IV tympanoplasty with overlay grafting, see Figs. **94A–C**. The type IV tympano-plasty is usually carried out in one stage in conjunction with an open mastoido-epitym-panectomy (see also mastoidectomy, p. 182).

Surgical Highlights

- General anesthesia
- Drilling of ponticulus to lower the tympanic sulcus to the level of oval window
- Anterior underlaid fascia covering round window, but leaving the oval window
- Oval window remains exposed
- Split-thickness skin grafting on stapes footplate

Surgical Steps

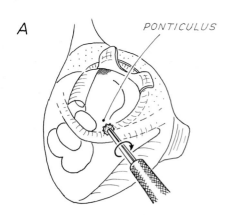

PONTICULUS

Fig. 41 A

Drilling of new tympanic sulcus

The new tympanic sulcus drilled over the ponticulus reaches the level of the oval window.

GELFILM

Fig. 41 B

Gelfilm sheeting of middle ear and eustachian tube

A Gelfilm sheet is placed in the hypotympanum and the proximal eustachian tube because of an active, chronic infection in the middle ear.

NEW TYMPANIC SULCUS

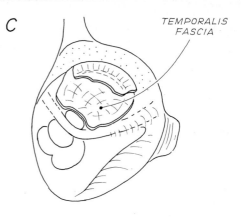

C

TEMPORALIS
FASCIA

Fig. **41 C**

Anterior underlay of temporalis fascia

The fresh temporalis fascia (see also Fig. 14 G) is placed under the anterior remnant of the drum and reaches the inferior border of the mobile footplate.

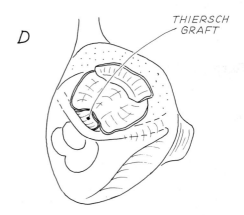

D

THIERSCH
GRAFT

Fig. **41 D**

Split-thickness skin grafting of the oval window

A split-thickness skin graft (Thiersch graft) is obtained from the posterior surface of the pinna with a No. 20 blade. The graft is placed over the footplate and kept in position by a Gelfoam pledget soaked in Ringer's solution.

b) Spandrel II

Surgical Technique

A Spandrel II is used for basic situation III₅ (mobile footplate, open cavity) in two stages. The Spandrel II is preferred to an autograft or biocompatible ossicle because of its better stability and superior hearing results. The first and last steps of the procedure are as for stapedotomy (see Figs. **107A–G**, pp. 215–17, and **116A–B**, pp. 226–7).

Surgical Highlights

- Local anesthesia
- Inferior tympanomeatal flap
- Spandrel with shoe and spike interposed between mobile footplate and undersurface of the drum

Surgical Steps

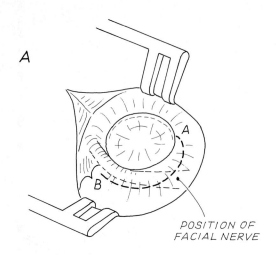

A

Fig. 42 A

Skin incision for inferior tympanomeatal flap

In open cavities, the skin incision for the tympanomeatal flap begins at 6 o'clock (*A*) and continues posterosuperiorly above the facial nerve (*B*). The skin incision is carried out superficially to avoid lesion of a possibly exposed facial nerve.

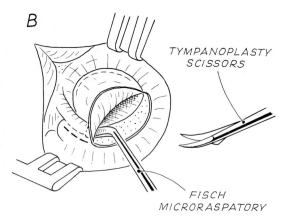

B

Fig. 42 B

Elevation of inferior tympanomeatal flap

The inferior tympanomeatal flap is elevated with a universal microraspatory. Expect a dehiscent facial nerve along the oval window niche. The "universal" microraspatory is an ideal instrument to elevate the tympanomeatal flap from the exposed facial nerve. The skin incision is extended superiorly with microscissors rather than with a knife to avoid a lesion of a possibly exposed facial nerve.

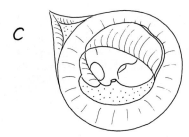

C

Fig. 42 C

Exposure of oval window niche

The mobile footplate is exposed. The tympanic facial nerve is dehiscent.

Fig. 42 D

Determination of the Spandrel's length

A malleable measuring rod is used to determine the distance between the mobile footplate and the tympanic membrane.

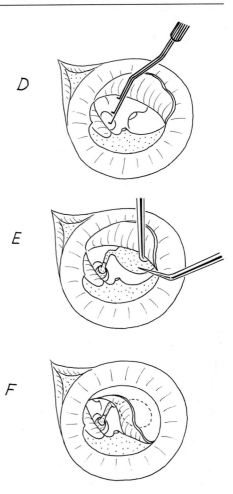

Fig. 42 E

Positioning of the Spandrel

The Spandrel is assembled as shown in Fig. 26 A–K. The Spandrel shoe with spike is placed over the mobile footplate. The Spandrel head is rotated bimanually under the center of the drum.

Fig. 42 F

Spandrel in position

The tympanomeatal flap should be elevated just enough to introduce the prosthesis, while leaving sufficient tension of the remaining drum to stabilize the Spandrel head.

c) Autograft or Biocompatible Ossicle

Surgical Technique

The functional results of an autograft or biocompatible ossicle are inferior to those of a Spandrel II (see results, p. 108). This may be a due to the less reliable stabilization of the ossicle. The operation is carried out at a second stage. The first and last steps are similar to those of stapedotomy (see Figs. **107A–G**, pp. 215–17, and **116A–B**, pp. 226–7).

Surgical Highlights

- Local anesthesia
- Inferior tympanomeatal flap
- Modified autograft ossicle between footplate and drum

Surgical Steps

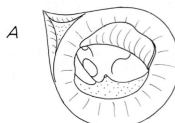

Fig. 43 A

Exposure of oval window niche

Surgical site with mobile footplate following elevation of tympanomeatal flap.

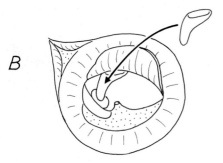

Fig. 43 B

Introduction of modified autograft incus

The autograft ossicle is prepared as shown in Figs. 28 A–D and then introduced between footplate and drum as for basic situation II (mobile footplate and malleus).

GELFOAM
+RINGER'S
SOLUTION

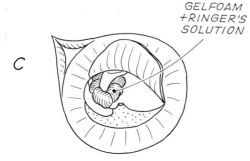

Fig. 43 C

Stabilization of the ossicle

The modified autograft incus is placed between the mobile footplate and drum. Gelfoam pledgets soaked in Ringer's solution and fibrin glue are used to stabilize the ossicle.

d) Neomalleus with Incus Replacement and Stapedotomy (NMIRS)

Surgical Technique

This procedure is carried out in two stages. The selection of patients is critical. Only ears without signs of tubal dysfunction for at least 6–12 months are eligible for this type of ossiculoplasty. The majority of neomalleus procedures are performed in patients who have had repeated failure of other types of reconstruction. The first and the last steps are carried out as for stapedotomy (see Figs. **107 A–G**, pp. 215–17, and **116A–B**, pp. 226–7).

Surgical Highlights

First Stage (Neomalleus, NM)

- Local anesthesia
- Inclusion of a modified autograft incus (or glass Ionomer ossicle [Ionos, Seefeld, Germany]) in the tragal perichondrium
- Underlay of perichondrium with neomalleus

Second Stage (Incus Replacement with Stapedotomy, IRS)

- Local anesthesia
- Identification and exposure of neomalleus
- Stapedotomy

Surgical Steps

First Stage (NM)

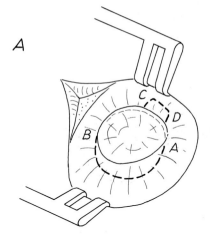

A

Fig. 44 A

Incision for tympanomeatal flaps

The skin incision for the superior tympanomeatal flap (*A–B*) is carried out between 7 o'clock and 12 o'clock. The rectangular anteroinferior tympanomeatal flap (*C–D*) is made between 4 o'clock and 5 o'clock (see Fig. 36 A–B).

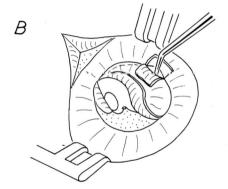

B

Fig. 44 B

Elevation of tympanomeatal flaps

When elevating the posteroinferior tympanomeatal flap, always expect an exposed or dehiscent facial nerve. Take care to preserve the tympanic annulus when elevating the tympanomeatal flaps.

C

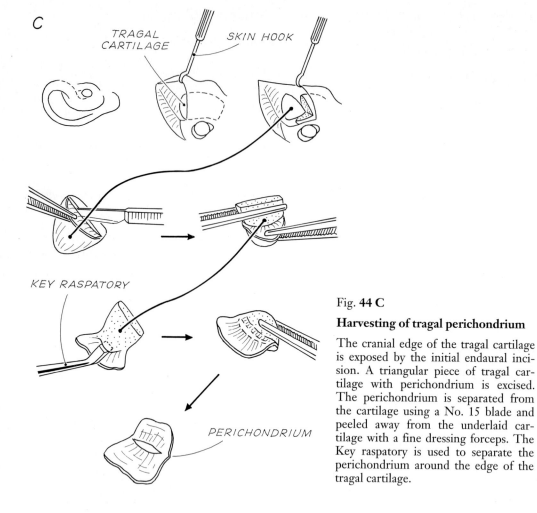

TRAGAL CARTILAGE

SKIN HOOK

KEY RASPATORY

PERICHONDRIUM

Fig. **44 C**

Harvesting of tragal perichondrium

The cranial edge of the tragal cartilage is exposed by the initial endaural incision. A triangular piece of tragal cartilage with perichondrium is excised. The perichondrium is separated from the cartilage using a No. 15 blade and peeled away from the underlaid cartilage with a fine dressing forceps. The Key raspatory is used to separate the perichondrium around the edge of the tragal cartilage.

D

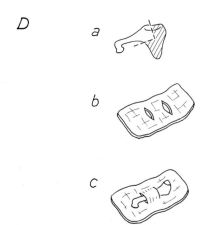

a

b

c

Fig. **44 D**

Inclusion of "neomalleus" in perichondrial graft

a: An autograft incus is modified to the shape of a "neomalleus".

b: Two incisions are made in the tragal perichondrium.

c: The "neomalleus" is inserted through the two incisions. The "neomalleus" can also be placed as shown in Fig. 36 D. Using an autograft ossicle carries the risk of resorption in the course of time. Using an Ionomer "neomalleus" (see Fig. 36 M–V) avoids this complication.

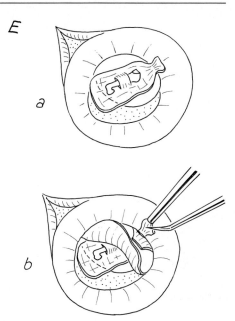

Fig. 44 E

Underlay of perichondrial graft with neomalleus

a: Schematic position of the underlaid graft with the long process of the incus over the oval window niche.

b: Actual underlay of the perichondrial graft showing the anterorinferior fixation between tympanic sulcus and annulus (see also Figs. 36 E, F, G).

Second Stage (IRS)

This surgery is carried out 3 to 6 months after the first stage if no signs of tubal dysfunction are present.

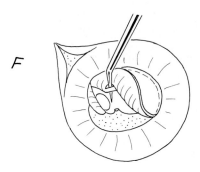

Fig. 44 F

Identification and exposure of the long process of the incus

The long process of the incus is separated from the surrounding soft tissues to allow attachment of the 0.4-mm TPP. In case of resorption of the autograft neomalleus, an Ionomer ossicle is modified as shown in Fig. 36 M–V.

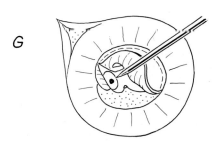

Fig. 44 G

Preparation of TPP and perforation of footplate

A 0.4-mm TPP is trimmed to the desired length on a cutting block. The proper length is verified in situ prior to stapedotomy. A 0.4-mm perforation is made through the mobile footplate using manual perforators (as for stapedotomy, see also Figs. 111 B–C, p. 221).

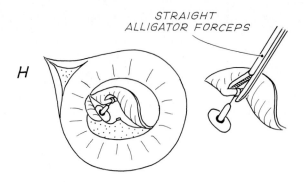

H

STRAIGHT
ALLIGATOR FORCEPS

Fig. **44 H**

Introduction and fixation of TPP

The 0.4-mm TPP is first attached to the exposed long process of the incus using fine alligator forceps. The Teflon piston is then introduced 0.5 mm into the vestibule.

5.3 Basic Situation III$_6$: Fixed Stapes, Open Cavity

This situation is managed using

a) Stapedectomy and Spandrel II, or
b) NMIRS.

a) Spandrel II with Stapedectomy

Surgical Technique

This operation is carried out as a second stage. The first and last steps of surgery are similar to those of stapedotomy (see Figs. **107 A–G**, pp. 215–17 and **116 A, B**, pp. 226–7).

Surgical Highlights

 Local anesthesia
● Total removal of footplate (stapedectomy)

- Perichondrium covering oval window
- Spandrel II with spike (but without shoe) between oval window and tympanic membrane

Surgical Steps

First Stage

The first-stage tympanoplasty is usually performed as a part of an open cavity (see p. 180).

Second Stage

The second-stage ossiculoplasty is performed 6–12 months later (see Figs. **31 A–I** and Figs. **37 A–D**). The operation is carried out only if there is no evidence of tubal dysfunction after the first surgery.

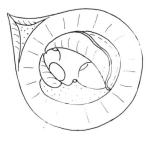

A

Fig. **45 A**

Elevation of the inferior tympanomeatal flap

The inferior tympanomeatal flap is raised, exposing the fixed footplate.

Fig. 45 B

Determination of prosthesis length and preparation of the Spandrel

A malleable measuring rod is used to determine the distance between the footplate and drum. The Spandrel is prepared with spike but without shoe as shown in Fig. 31 D–I, pp. 66,67).

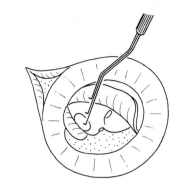

B

Fig. 45 C

Total removal of footplate (stapedectomy)

The fixed footplate is removed in two halves as in stapedectomy (see Fig. 118 G–H, p. 229).

C

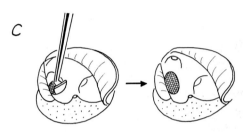

Fig. 45 D

Tragal perichondrium over oval window

Tragal perichondrium is used to cover the open the oval window (see Fig. 31 B–C, p.65).

D

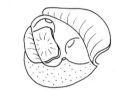

Fig. 45 E

Introduction of the Spandrel

The Spandrel without shoe is picked up with a large microsuction tube and introduced with its spike into the center of the oval window. The prosthesis head is then rotated bimanually under the tympanic membrane.

E

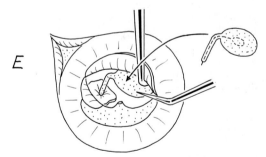

F

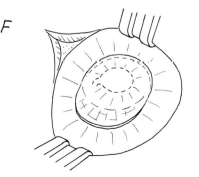

Fig. 45 F

Final position of the Spandrel

The broken line shows the final position of the Spandrel head after replacement of the tympanomeatal flap.

b) Neomalleus with Incus Replacement and Stapedotomy (NMIRS)

The ossiculoplasty is carried out as shown for basic situation III-5 (mobile footplate, open cavity, Figs. **44A–H**). A special type of TPP, 4 mm long and 0.4 mm in diameter (Xomed Treace) has been developed to cope with the shallow cavum tympani of an open cavity.

6. Factors that Improve the Results of Ossicular Reconstruction

The functional results of ossiculoplasty are improved by

1. Epitympanectomy
2. Middle ear and eustachian tube sheeting
3. Reconstruction of posterosuperior canal wall and reinforcement of posterosuperior tympanic membrane
4. Transmastoid drainage
5. Staging

6.1 Epitympanectomy

Indication. Irreversible disease in the attic.

Rationale. Removal of the chorda–tensor fold and malleus head improves ventilation of the anterior attic. In normal ears, the anterior attic is a separate compartment with critical ventilation. A pathological change of the mucosal lining of the attic interferes with the adequate ventilation of the anterior epitympanum and may induce retractions of the Shrapnell membrane (see also Pathogenesis of medial attic cholesteatoma, Fig. **74**, p. 148). Analysis of 30 normal temporal bones has shown that the chorda–tensor fold is closed in two-thirds of the cases and presents a small opening for ventilation of the anterior attic in one-third of the specimens (Fig. **46**).

Epitympanectomy: This comprises removing the incus and malleus head (including the superior malleolar fold) and exposing the entire attic (see Fig. **47**). All bony overhangs are removed with the burr. The chorda–tensor fold is carefully removed so as to create a large communication between the tympanic ostium of the eustachian tube and the anterior attic. The cellular tracts situated superior to the tensor muscle *(supratubal recess)* as well as the pneumatic cells situated between the tympanic segment of the facial nerve, the lateral and superior ampullae, and the middle cranial fossa dura *(supralabyrinthine recess)* should be exenterated. The attachment of the tensor tympani tendon to the malleus should be preserved.

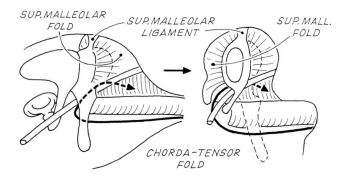

A) The chorda-tensor fold is closed in 2/3 of cases

Fig. 46

Chorda–tensor fold in normal ears

A: In normal ears, the anterior attic (epitympanum) is a nearly closed space with critical ventilation. In two-thirds of the cases, the chorda–tensor fold is closed, and ventilation of the attic is provided from the tympanic isthmus through a small opening in the superior malleolar fold.

B: In one-third of the cases, the anterior attic is ventilated through an opening in the chorda–tensor fold.

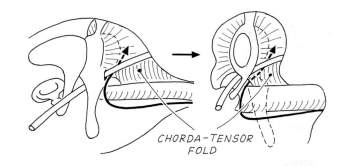

B) The chorda-tensor fold is open in 1/3 of cases

A: Mastoidectomy, posterior
tympanotomy

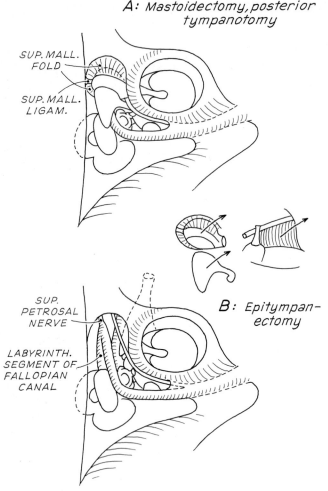

SUP. MALL.
FOLD

SUP. MALL.
LIGAM.

SUP.
PETROSAL
NERVE

LABYRINTH.
SEGMENT OF
FALLOPIAN
CANAL

B: Epitympan-
ectomy

Fig. **47**

Epitympanectomy

A: View of the attic following mastoidectomy, posterior tympanotomy, and removal of the lateral attic wall.

B: The epitympanectomy comprises the removal of the incus, of the malleus head, and of the chorda–tensor fold. The supratubal and supralabyrinthine cells are exenterated as much as possible. A complete exenteration of the supratubal and supralabyrinthine cell tracts is only possible in open cavities.

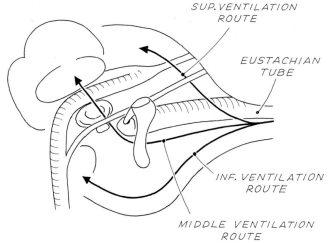

SUP. VENTILATION
ROUTE

EUSTACHIAN
TUBE

INF. VENTILATION
ROUTE

MIDDLE VENTILATION
ROUTE

Fig. **48**

Ventilation routes of the attic after epitympanectomy (closed cavity)

Removal of the incus, malleus head, and chorda–tensor fold has reestablished the *superior ventilation route* to the anterior attic, which is essential for preventing retractions of the superior drum. The *middle ventilation route* reaches the posterior attic through the tympanic isthmus. The *inferior ventilation route* to the round window niche is along the hypotympanum.

6.2 Middle Ear and Eustachian Tube Sheeting

a) Indication

The indications for sheeting with thick
(1 mm) Silastic (Dow Corning, see instru-
mentation) or Gelfilm (Ethicon) are:
– Raw surface of middle ear mucosa
– Poor eustachian tube function
– Stapes only (no incus and malleus)

b) Shaping

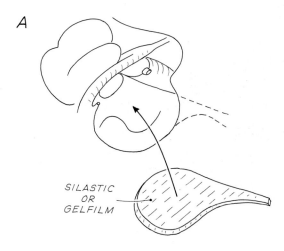

A

SILASTIC
OR
GELFILM

Fig. **49**

B

**Shape of middle ear and eustachian tube
sheets**

A: The Silastic (1 mm) or Gelfilm sheets are
fashioned to fill the entire middle ear cavity
and to extend into the tympanic ostium toward
the isthmus of the eustachian tube.

B: Sheeting in place

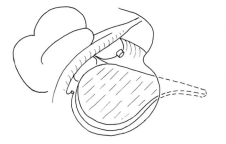

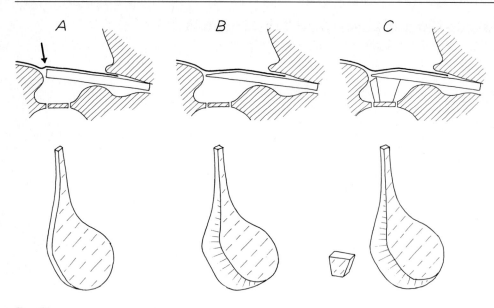

Fig. **50**

Shaping of Silastic sheets

A: Sharp edges of the thick (1 mm) Silastic sheet must be avoided because of possible perforation of the new drum.

B: Sharp edges of the Silastic sheet are eliminated by cutting away the excess material with curved tympanoplasty scissors.

C: A small piece of the Silastic sheet can be placed between the main sheet and the mobile footplate. This prevents scar formation and provides some degree of sound transmission while waiting for the second-stage ossiculoplasty.

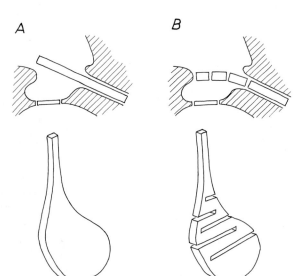

Fig. **51**

Alternate cuts to reduce rigidity of thick (1 mm) Silastic sheeting

A: The angulation between the middle ear and eustachian tube may not allow proper fitting of the Silastic sheeting.

B: Alternate cuts in the Silastic sheeting reduce the rigidity of the material and allow adequate adaptation in the middle ear cavity.

6.3 Reconstruction of the Posterosuperior Canal Wall and Reinforcement of the Drum

a) Use of Septal Cartilage

Septal cartilage, preserved in 4% Formalin for 2 weeks and then in a solution of 1:5000 mercury compound (Cialit), is placed in Ringer's solution at least 30 minutes before use. The cartilage is cut to the proper size and shaped with a knife. Cross-etching is used to reduce stiffness when needed.

Fig. 52

Reconstruction of postero-superior canal wall with septal cartilage

A: In ears with extensive destruction of the ossicular chain, the lateral wall of the attic is usually atrophic.

B: A slice of preserved septal cartilage is placed over the posterosuperior canal wall. The preserved septal cartilage is supported by the Silastic sheeting placed into the middle ear. If the cartilage is too rigid, cross-etchings are made with a knife on its surface in order to obtain proper plasticity.

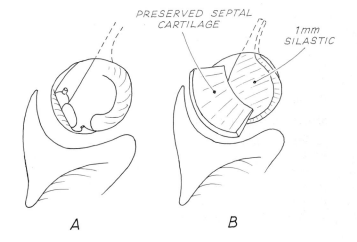

PRESERVED SEPTAL CARTILAGE

1mm SILASTIC

A   B

b) Use of Tragal Cartilage and Perichondrium

Cartilage obtained from the tragus is an alternative for reconstruction of the posterosuperior canal wall.

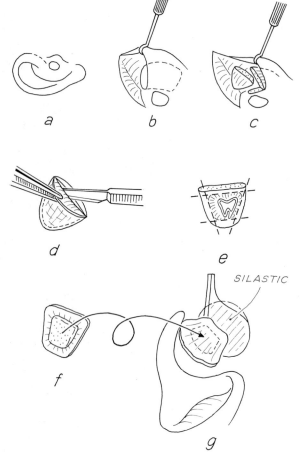

Fig. **53**

Reconstruction of posterosuperior canal wall with tragal cartilage and perichondrium

a: The endaural incision exposes the cranial end of the tragal cartilage.

b, c: A triangular piece of tragal cartilage is cut away.

d: The perichondrium is elevated from one side of the cartilage and left attached to the opposite side.

e: The cartilage is cut to the desired size.

f: Cartilage ready for use.

g: For reconstruction of the posterosuperior canal wall, the cartilage is placed medially, and the perichondrial flap stabilizes the reconstructed canal wall on its lateral surface.

c) Use of Conchal Cartilage and Perichondrium

The use of cartilage from the concha is an alternative to tragal cartilage.

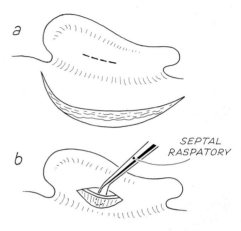

Fig. **54**

Reconstruction of the posterosuperior canal wall with conchal cartilage and perichondrium

a: An incision is made behind the pinna at the level of the conchal cartilage.

b: The conchal cartilage is incised and the skin elevated from the opposite side using a septal raspatory.

c, d, e: The resected cartilage is cut to the desired size.

f: The cartilage on the reconstructed canal wall is stabilized with the perichondrium.

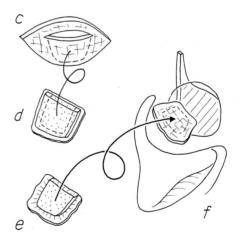

d) Use of Bone from the Temporal Squama

The posterosuperior canal wall can be reconstructed using a bone flap from the temporal squama.

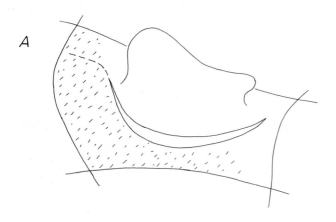

A

Fig. 55 A

Skin incision

The retroauricular skin incision is extended superiorly over the temporal squama.

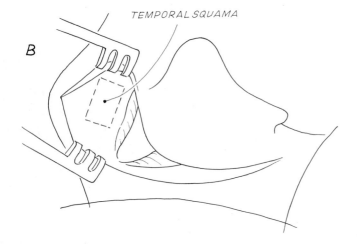

B

TEMPORAL SQUAMA

Fig. 55 B

Exposure of temporal squama

The temporalis muscle is elevated with a retroauricular retractor, exposing the temporal squama above the temporal line.

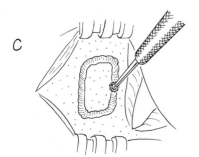

C

Fig. 55 C

Removal of bone flap

A 2 × 1-cm bone flap is removed using a 5-mm cutting burr on a straight handpiece and suction irrigation. A 4-mm diamond burr is used to remove the last shell of bone to avoid damaging the dura or branches of the middle meningeal artery.

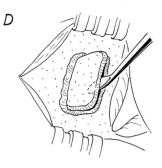

Fig. 55 D

Elevation of bone flap

A septal raspatory is used to elevate the bone flap from the dura.

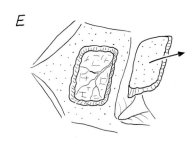

Fig. 55 E

Surgical site after removal of bone flap

Bleeding from small dural branches of the middle meningeal artery is stopped with bipolar coagulation.

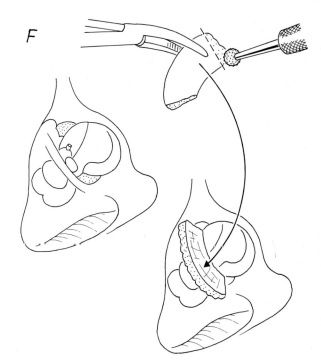

Fig. 55 F

Shaping of bone flap and reconstruction of posterosuperior canal wall

The size of the bone flap is reduced with a diamond burr as needed. The lateral margins of the flap are cut in an oblique plane to obtain the necessary stabilization. The reconstructed canal wall can be supported by an additional piece of bone (Fig. 79 C), bone paste (bone dust and fibrin glue), or bioglass cement (Ionos, see instrumentation).

6.4 Transmastoid Drainage

The transmastoid drain (Kaja drain) is used in a closed cavity whenever the eustachian tube function is questionable and an antrotomy has been performed (see also Fig. **18 D–F**, p. 36). The drain is introduced through a separate retroauricular incision. Polyethylene tubing with an outer diameter of 5 mm is used. The tubing has been permanently bent by placing it over a curved metal stylus and heating it in an oven at a temperature of 80 °C. The angle of the bend is 110°. Alternatively, a Silastic tube may be used. A suction tube of a smaller diameter than the internal diameter of the drain is used daily after surgery to remove fluid accumulating in the antrum. The drain is removed when fluid production has ceased and/or the Valsalva maneuver has become positive (usually 4 to 8 days postoperative).

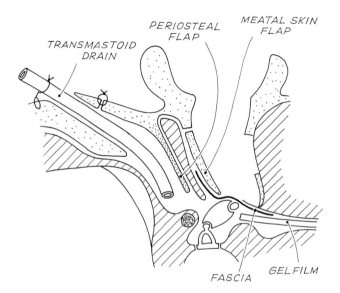

Fig. **56**

Transmastoid drainage

Schematic view of the surgical site after wound closure. The transmastoid drain is introduced through a separate retroauricular incision and fixed in place with a 2–0 silk suture. The retroauricular periosteal flap covers the posterior canal wall and should prevent postoperative atrophy of the latter. The figure shows the situation in the middle ear following an anterior underlaid fascial graft with one-stage incus interposition.

6.5 Staging

Reconstruction of the ossicular chain is best performed 6 months to 1 year after restoration of an aerated middle ear cavity to ensure ideal position and stability of the sound transformer mechanism, particularly of the drum.

In cases of extensive ossicular destruction, the stapes arch is often fixed to the promontory. Removal of the arch increases mobility of the footplate and improves functional results.

Rationale

Staging permits
– Stabilization of the drum
– Regrowth of the mucosal lining of the middle ear,
– Evaluation of the ventilating efficiency of the eustachian tube

Fig. **57**

Closed cavity: schematic representation after first-stage tympanoplasty

A thick Silastic sheet was placed in the middle ear and the eustachian tube. The posterior canal wall was reconstructed with septal cartilage. The underlaid fascia is supported anteriorly by the Silastic sheeting. The meatal skin flap covers the posterior fascia. The inner surface of the posterior canal wall is covered by the mastoid periosteal flap to reduce the danger of postoperative bone atrophy and to avoid ingrowth of meatal skin in the mastoid.

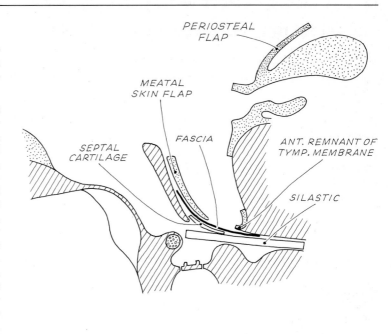

Fig. **58**

Open cavity: schematic representation after first-stage tympanoplasty

Thick Silastic sheeting with alternate cuts (see Fig. 51) is introduced into the middle ear and eustachian tube. The Silastic sheeting supports the underlaid fascia against the undersurface of the anterior remnant of the drum and surrounding bone. Reepithelization of the anterior canal wall proceeds from the meatal skin and the anterior tympanomeatal flap.

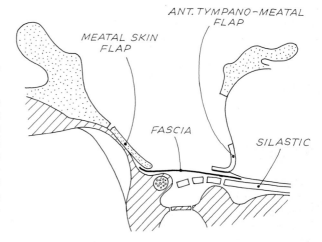

7. Results of Ossiculoplasty

It is clear that the subjective benefit of ossiculoplasty depends on the binaural hearing ability of the patient. Therefore, the air–bone gap alone is an insufficient measure of the hearing gain experienced by an individual patient. When advising ossiculoplasty to a patient, the surgeon should consider the condition of the opposite ear, with particular attention to the criteria advocated by Smyth and Patterson (the operated ear better than 30 dB or within 15 dB of the other ear).

From a technical point of view, the closure of the air–bone gap still remains the best indicator of the success of a specific ossicular reconstruction. With this information, the surgeon should be able to predict the possible hearing gain achievable in a patient.

The selection of a particular method of ossiculoplasty depends on three criteria:

1. The method should give better results than another
2. The method should be simpler and therefore more economical in time than another
3. With equivalent results, the more economical method should be preferred

Table 4 reviews the first choice for ossiculoplasty as it relates to the different conditions of the ossicular chain presented in this manual. Stapedotomy with a postoperative average air–bone gap of 0–10 dB remains the "gold standard" of ossiculoplasty. The results for all other ossicular reconstructions fall short of those of stapedotomy. Incus interposition, IRS, and NMIRS achieve the second best results with an expected average air–bone gap of 10–20 dB. The reconstruction with Spandrel II comes next with an average postoperative air–bone gap of 20–30 dB. The type III tympanoplasty yields on average the least satisfactory postoperative air–bone gap of 30–40 dB. These figures, obtained with long-term follow-up (5 years to 10 years) give an important indication of the *limitation* inherent in a particular ossicular situation. It is logical to expect that postoperative hearing is related to the loss of ossicular tissue. This is reflected by the fact that the reconstruction of the *missing incus* gives an air–bone gap that is 20 dB better than the columella reconstruction of the *stapes only* situation. The incus interposition gives results that are 10 dB less than those of stapedotomy. This shows the importance of the incudomalleolar complex for sound transmission. Differences of 10 dB may seem minimal; however, these "small" variations in functional outcome may have a tremendous impact on the hearing benefit of the patient, particularly considering the function of the opposite ear.

Table 4   Hearing results of various types of ossiculoplasty. The expected range of the postoperative air–bone gap is defined by the 10 dB range in which the hearing of the majority of the patients was found 3 years postoperatively

Type of ossiculoplasty	Basic situation of ossicular Chain	Expected range of postoperative air–bone gap
Stapedotomy		0–10 dB
Incusinterposition	I	10–20 dB
Incus replacement and stapedotomy	II	10–20 dB
Neomalleus with incus replacement and stapedotomy	II	10–20 dB
Spandrel	III	20–30 dB
Type III tympanoplasty	III	30–40 dB

Through the years, we have come to the conclusion that the limitations imposed by the condition of the ossicular tissues have been underestimated. The results obtained by columella reconstructions are all equivalent in the long term. Better results of the *stapes only* situation are probably not achievable with any new biocompatible material or any new shape of prosthesis. A real advance in the results of ossiculoplasty is possible by converting an unfavorable basic ossicular situation to a more favorable one (e. g. a basic situation III to a basic situation II). The limitations exhibited by the results obtained with Spandrel II demonstrate this need.

One of our goals in ossiculoplasty has been to develop a columella prosthesis, the Spandrel II, capable of reproducing the action of the incudomalleolar joint by means of an angulated wire core. A recent dynamic and natural frequency analysis using the finite element method by Williams (1992) has shown that the Spandrel II works more efficiently in collecting and transmitting sound to the stapes footplate than a more rigid prosthesis. Accordingly, the Spandrel II has given rewarding functional results in the stapes only situation. However, we were unable to close the average air–bone gap better than 20–30 dB in the long term. Because of these results, we have chosen to convert selected cases of basic situation III (stapes only) into a more favorable situation II (malleus and stapes) by incorporating a neomalleus into the tympanic membrane. A subsequent stapedotomy with introduction of 0.4-mm TPP between the new malleus and the vestibule has allowed closure of the air–bone gap to within 10–20 dB. The neomalleus procedure avoids the difficulty found in stabilization of the prosthesis to the drum and the footplate of a columella reconstruction. A drawback of the neomalleus procedure is the possibility of a sensorineural hearing loss as in surgery for otosclerotic ears. This is why the Spandrel II reconstruction and the type III tympanoplasty are still indicated, particularly in children who may have unstable eustachian tube function.

Table 5 shows the average air–bone gap reached at the end of a 3-year follow-up by different types of ossicular reconstruction. The limitations of the different techniques are clearly visible. The only technique permitting an air–bone closure within 0–20 dB in 79% of the cases was stapedotomy. Incus interposition, IRS, and NMIRS obtained the same air–bone closure in 59% of the cases. The Spandrel II and type III tympanoplasty yield an equal result in 25% and 23% of the patients. These general results have not changed at 5-year and 10-year follow-up (see also Fig. 59). However, it will take a few years longer before we have sufficient data to present the 10-year results of the Spandrel II and neomalleus procedure.

Table 5   Hearing results vs. type of ossicular reconstruction (3-year follow-up)

Air–bone gap (dB)	Stapedotomy (n = 330)	Incus interp. (n = 22)	Incus repl. + staped. (n = 24)	Neomalleus + IRS (n = 23)	Spandrel (n = 28)	Type III (n = 26)
0–10	52%	27%	25%	–	7%	–
0–20	79%	54%	58%	64%	32%	23%
0–30	88%	91%	85%	91%	61%	69%
> 30	12%	9%	15%	9%	39%	31%

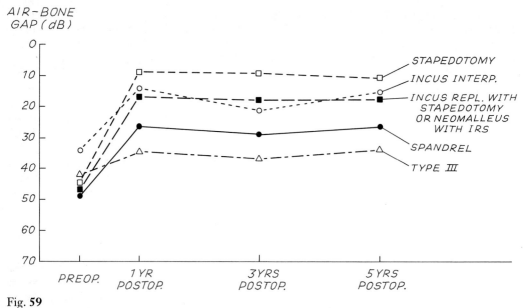

AIR–BONE GAP (dB)

STAPEDOTOMY
INCUS INTERP.
INCUS REPL. WITH STAPEDOTOMY OR NEOMALLEUS WITH IRS
SPANDREL
TYPE III

PREOP.   1 YR POSTOP.   3 YRS POSTOP.   5 YRS POSTOP.

Fig. 59

Long-term results of techniques of ossiculo-plasty

This is a graphic representation of the results obtained in ossicular reconstruction with the various techniques illustrated in this manual. There is a remarkable stability of the results over time. In the following pages, the functional results of each type of ossiculoplasty are discussed in detail.

7.1 Incus Interposition

Table 6 shows the 5- and 10-year follow-up results of incus interposition. In spite of favorable conditions for ossicular reconstruction, only 54% and 60%, respectively of the patients closed the air–bone gap within 0–20 dB as also shown in Tables 4 and 5 and

Fig. **59**. The finding that incus interposition is unable to achieve equivalent results to stapedotomy is probably due to the bypass of the incudomalleal complex. This complex must play a primary role in conferring the combination of rigidity and flexibility necessary for optimum sound conduction to the ossicular chain and for the continuous com-

Table **6**   Long-term results of incus interposition (n = 55)

Air–bone gap (dB)	Preoperative		Postoperative 5 years		10 years	
	n	(%)	n	(%)	n	(%)
0–10	–	(–)	7	(25)	3	(20)
0–20	6	(11)	15	(54)	9	(60)
0–30	25	(45)	25	(89)	13	(87)
>30	30	(55)	3	(11)	2	(13)
Total	55	(100)	28	(100)	15	(100)

pliance to the changes in position of the tympanic membrane.

The long-term results of incus interposition* show (Fig. **59**) that the maximum hearing gain is already achieved within 3 months following surgery. The use of a biocompatible glass Ionomer ossicle has given similar results to those obtained with homologous ossicles.

7.2 Incus Replacement with Stapedotomy (IRS)

This technique has been used increasingly in the past 5 years. The ideal indication is a mobile or fixed footplate with malleus handle and intact anterior tympanic membrane (basic situation II). Only patients without signs of tubal dysfunction for at least 6–12 months preoperatively are selected for IRS. The 3-year and 5–year follow-up results are shown in Table **5** and Fig. **59**.

The closure of the air–bone gap equals that obtained with incus interposition. No total or partial sensorineural loss has been recorded to date, even in patients with severe postoperative retraction of the tympanic membrane. Therefore, the fixation of the 0.4–mm TPP adjacent to the lateral process

---

* Schmid S, Fisch U, Gürtler Th. In: Charachon R, Garcia-Ibanez E, eds. Long Term Results and Indications in Otology and Otoneurosurgery, Amsterdam: Kugler Ghedini, 1991.

of the malleus handle should offer effective protection to the inner ear when the malleus handle is retracted by negative pressure in the middle ear (see Fig. **24 H**, p. 53).

IRS has been used in conjunction with a mobile footplate in trauma (particularly traumatic rupture of the stapes arch) and in chronic otitis media with destruction of the stapes arch. Patients selected for IRS should not present with signs of eustachian tube dysfunction for 6–12 months before surgery. Patients with perforated tympanic membranes are treated in two stages.

7.3 Spandrel II

In our experience, the Spandrel II has proven the best available columellar prosthesis. In the first edition of this book (1980), we reported that TORPs gave superior results to homologous ossicles; Figs. **59**, **60** and **61** show that the Spandrel II yields better closure of the air–bone gap than the type III tympanoplasty in the long term. The stability of the results achieved with Spandrel II over time is remarkable (Table **7**). No differences in hearing results were observed with Spandrel II in open and closed cavities (Fig. **61**).

Figs. **60** and **61** show that the average air–bone gap was improved from 50 dB (preoperative) to 25–30 dB (postoperative). Using the Smith and Patterson criteria (operated ear better than 30 dB or within 15 dB of the other ear), the Spandrel II opera-

Table **7** Hearing results of Spandrel

Hearing level	Preop.		1 year postop.		3 years postop.		5 years postop.	
(AC, dB)	n	(%)	n	(%)	n	(%)	n	(%)
0–20	–	(–)	–	(–)	–	(–)	–	(–)
0–30	1	(2)	7	(13)	2	(7)	2	(18)
0–40	2	(4)	21	(39)	8	(29)	4	(36)
0–50	7	(13)	33	(61)	12	(43)	6	(55)
0–60	8	(15)	42	(80)	19	(68)	10	(91)
>60	44	(85)	10	(20)	9	(32)	1	(9)

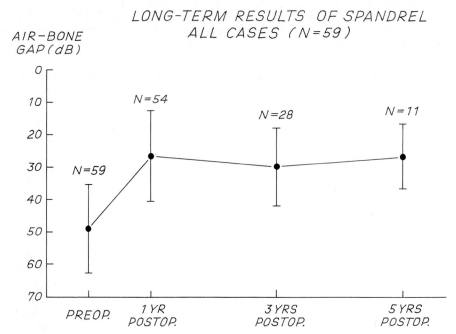

Fig. **60**

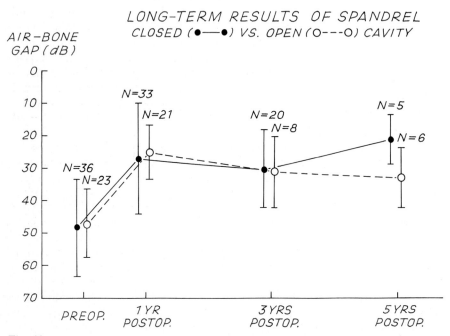

Fig. **61**

tion would have benefited only 7–8% of the patients with normal contralateral ears. On the other hand, 43%–55% of the patients with a contralateral hearing loss of 30–40 dB would have been satisfied with the operation. This shows that the Spandrel II can be of reasonable help to a patient with bilateral hearing problems.

The *extrusion* rate of Spandrel II in the first 5 years has been 4.5%. The number of extrusions is remarkably low when one considers that the head of the Spandrel II was not protected by cartilage or other material. Apparently, the angulation of the wire core provides sufficient elasticity to comply with the movement of the tympanic membrane when swallowing, sneezing, and changing altitude.

A previous study on TORPs (Table **8**) demonstrated that the lowest rate of extrusion (3.3%) was found in the presence of an intact tympanic membrane and a normal eustachian tube. The highest rate of extrusion (21%) occurred in open cavities with poor eustachian tube function. These facts emphasize the importance of eustachian tube function in the selection of patients for columellar reconstructions. For the same reason, patients requiring both myringoplasty and columellar reconstruction should be staged.

7.4 Neomalleus with Incus Replacement and Stapedotomy (NMIRS)

The neomalleus with incus replacement and stapedotomy (NMIRS) was developed to convert a less favorable ossicular situation (basic situation III: stapes only) into a more favorable one (basic situation II: malleus handle and stapes footplate). The disadvantage of NMIRS is the possible danger of a sensorineural hearing loss. In 49 patients who have undergone surgery since 1988, no total or partial postoperative sensorineural hearing loss has been observed.

Fig. **62** shows a detailed analysis of the 3-year follow-up of the first 12 patients who un-

Table **8** Extrusion rate of TORPs in various types of ossicular reconstructions (n = 132)

Total incidence	8/132	(6%)
Extrusion vs. type of surgery		
One stage (intact drum, normal ET function)	1/30	(3.3%)
Staged (all cases)	7/102	(6.9%)
Staged (wall up)	2/44	(4.5%)
Staged (wall down)	5/24	(21%)

derwent surgery with NMIRS. All patients had a bilateral severe conductive hearing loss and were operated on 3–7 times (average 4.5 times) previously (homologous ossicles, ceramic TORPs, cartilage struts, etc.) without success. NMIRS has yielded a hearing improvement of 20–50 dB in all cases. Seven out of 12 patients (58%) reached a hearing threshold within 25–30 dB. The other 5 patients were subjectively pleased about their hearing benefits, which allowed them to successfully wear a hearing aid.

The majority of the patients with NMIRS had a two-stage procedure. Only patients with normal eustachian tube function were selected for surgery. In four instances (8%), the operation had to be repeated 6 months to a year later because of migration of the prosthesis. The recurrent conductive hearing loss was caused by the lateralization of the drum and neomalleus. We have learned that the autograft incus can be resorbed within a year. We have, therefore, started to use Ionomer ossicles (see instrumentation) for the neomalleus. This has eliminated the problem of resorption and reduced postoperative migration of the neomalleus considerably.

Fig. **63** shows a comparison between preoperative and postoperative (1–3 years) results of Spandrel II and NMIRS. On average, the hearing threshold after the NMIRS was 10 dB better than with the Spandrel II. This is a tremendous advantage for patients because the operation provides a hearing bene-

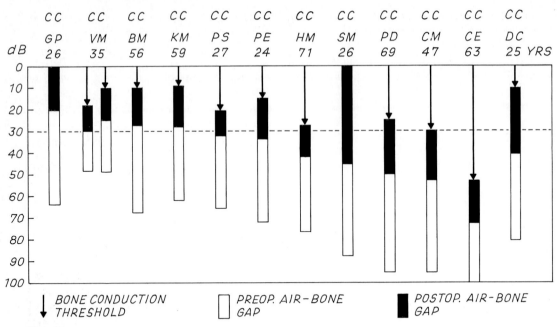

Fig. **62**

Results of neomalleus stapedotomy (N = 12)

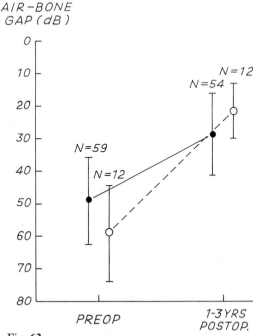

Fig. **63**

Results of neomalleus stapedotomy (○——○) vs. Spandrel (●–●)

fit even in the presence of normal contralateral hearing. This is why we continue to use the neomalleus procedure.

7.5 Type III Tympanoplasty

Type III tympanoplasty consists of placing the drum over the head of the mobile stapes. This is the only one-stage ossicular reconstruction that we perform systematically in open cavities. The decision to use a one-stage type III tympanoplasty rather than a two-stage TORP is based on the finding that there is no significant difference between the techniques after long-term follow-up. In adults, no statistical difference was found in the hearing gain 3 years postoperatively after type III tympanoplasty (open cavity) and TORPs (closed cavity) (Table **9**). The prerequisite for a good functional result in type III tympanoplasty is the formation of a new bony sulcus lower than the head of the stapes. The results of type III tympanoplasty compared to those of Spandrel II in adults are shown in Table **5**. Fewer patients attained an air–bone gap of 0–20 dB at 3-year follow-up with type III tympanoplasty than with

Table **9** Hearing results in open and closed cavity for TORPs and tympanoplasty type III (Three-year follow up)

Air-Bone Gap (dB)	closed cavity (TORP, n = 55)		open cavity (Type III, n = 26)	
	n	(%)	n	(%)
0–10	–	(–)	1	(4)
0–20	9	(17)	6	(23)
0–30	30	(55)	18	(69)
>30	25	(45)	8	(31)

Spandrel II. However, there was no substantial difference between the groups in the number of patients who attained an air–bone gap of 0–30 dB.

The results of type III tympanoplasty and TORPs were investigated in children by Schmid et al. (1991)* 5 years and 10 years fol-

---

* Schmid H, Dort JC, Fisch U. Am J Oto 1991; 2: 83–87.

lowing surgery (Table **10**). The residual air–bone gap after type III tympanoplasty was slightly better than that following a two-stage TORP in an open cavity after 10 years. No statistical difference was found at the 10-year follow-up between type III tympanoplasty and two-stage TORP (22 dB and 20 dB, respectively) in closed cavities.

In adults, no statistical difference was found in the hearing gain 3 years after type III tympanoplasty (open cavity) and TORPs (closed cavity) (see Table 9).

7.6 Results of Epitympanectomy

The important role of the attic and, particularly, of the anterior epitympanic space is well supported by the fact that the number of posterosuperior or attic retraction pockets observed following systematic epitympanectomy is considerably less than that seen when the malleus head has been left in place.

Table **10** Hearing results of ossiculoplasty in children. Stapes only in open (Basic Situation III$_4$) and closed cavity (Basic Situation III$_1$)

	Hearing level in dB		
	Preop.	5 years postop.	10 years postop.
Type III (one stage, open cavity)	(n = 11)	(n = 4)	(n = 7)
AC	40 (± 12)	46 (± 17)	31 (± 19)
BC	2	9	9
A–B gap	38	37	22
TORP (2 stages, open cavity)	(n = 5)	(n = 2)	(n = 3)
AC	47 (± 14.5)	58 (± 4.2)	55 (± 15.9)
BC	3	24	25
A–B gap	44	34	30
TORP (2 stages, closed cavity)	(n = 6)	(n = 3)	(n = 3)
AC	46 (± 20)	38 (± 19)	35 (± 5)
BC	14	11	15
A–B gap	32	27	20

The figures presented in Table **11** were obtained in patients who underwent surgery for chronic otitis media or atelectatic ears without cholesteatoma. We do not have a similar comparative study for cholesteatoma because, as a result of the investigations of Rüedi, systematic epitympanectomy has always been performed when the cholesteatoma involved the attic (see p. 148).

The limited number of recurrent or residual cholesteatoma observed in the closed cavities of our patients (see p. 194) must be attributed to the prevention of attic disease induced by poor ventilation as well as to the facilitation of the removal of the matrix from the anterior attic afforded by systematic epitympanectomy.

Table **11** Localization of retraction pockets following intact canal technique (3-year follow-up, n = 126)

Type of surgery	Posterosuperior or attic retraction	
	n	%
Malleus head in place	18/75	24.0
Systematic epitympanectomy	4/51	7.8

8. Rules and Hints

- Incus interposition gives results that are on average 10 dB less than those of stapedotomy.
- Stage reconstruction of the ossicular chain whenever the malleus handle is absent.
- Patients will accept staged surgery if they know that this will offer them a better hearing result and that the second stage is performed under local anesthesia without hospitalization.
- Wait 6–12 months for the second-stage operation in order to obtain stabilization of the drum, epithelization of the middle ear cavity, and assessment of tubal function.
- The anterior attic has a critical ventilation, and the tensor–chorda fold is the key to its ventilation.
- Perform epitympanectomy whenever irreversible disease in the mastoid and attic is present.
- Knowledge of the anatomy of the labyrinthine segment of the facial nerve is essential when the supralabyrinthine and apical cellular tracts must be exenterated.
- Use thick Silastic sheeting when reepithelization of rough surfaces in the middle ear is needed.
- Use Gelfilm sheeting rather than Silastic in chronically infected ears.
- Thick Silastic sheets help in anterior underlay grafting by permitting easy introduction of the underlaid fascial graft and keeping it in contact with the lateral wall of the middle ear cavity.
- Reinforce the posterosuperior canal wall and posterosuperior quadrant of the drum with cartilage whenever atrophy of the bone is present.
- Septal or tragal cartilage will not fix to the bony rim of the external canal but rather incorporates into the surrounding tissue.
- Positioning of the retroauricular periosteal flap on the preserved posterior canal wall prevents atrophy of bone and invasion of the meatal epithelium into the mastoid.
- Use transmastoid drainage in the presence of insufficient eustachian tube function.
- The transmastoid drainage helps clear postoperative secretions and ensures proper ventilation of the middle ear.
- Place Spandrel II over the footplate, even in the presence of stapedial arch.
- Remove stapedial arch with crurotomy scissors whenever it is fixed to the promontory.
- Use pressed tragal perichondrium to seal the oval window when stapedectomy is necessary.
- If performed in a second-stage ossiculoplasty, stapedotomy on a mobile footplate is no more dangerous than in otosclerosis.

- Use the chorda tympani to stabilize the modified ossicle in incus interposition.
- Cutting the tensor tympani tendon will reduce the stability of incus interposition.
- Check the proper size of a Spandrel, ossicle, or prosthesis by placing it in situ. Be prepared to make successive adjustment to the size and length.
- If a perforation occurs in the presence of Silastic sheeting in the middle ear, a chronic foreign body reaction will occur requiring removal.
- Ionomer ossicles are more fragile than human ossicles and require special care when grasping with the clamp for shaping.
- In incus replacement with stapedotomy, expose the lateral process and adjacent malleus handle to avoid difficult introduction and crimping of the prosthesis through a tunnel.
- Use a manual perforator when making the stapedotomy in a mobile footplate. This instrument has the advantage of allowing one to "feel" the amount of pressure exerted by the tip. This is in contrast to an electric microdrill.
- In incus replacement with stapedotomy, it is essential to attach the prosthesis close to the lateral process of the malleus to avoid large movements of the piston into the vestibule.
- Spandrel II differs from Spandrel I by the central position of the wire platform, a thinner polycel head, and the wire core protruding from the shoe (spike).
- The ability to flex the head of the Spandrel II avoids the necessity of tissue coverage to avoid extrusion.
- In Spandrel II, or similar columellar struts, the tympanomeatal flap should be raised just enough to allow placement of the prosthesis while preserving sufficient tension of the remaining drum for its fixation.
- In wide oval window niches, extra stabilization of the shoe of the Spandrel II can be obtained with small pieces of tragal cartilage.
- When trimming the shaft of the Spandrel II, avoid damaging the casing by grasping the shaft at the point where the polycel is to be cut. Use a No. 11 blade to make a clean circumferential cut in the polycel casing before removing the excess from the wire core.
- The Spandrel shoe can be reduced in size to allow it to fit between the stapes crura.
- The properly fitted Spandrel II should produce a slight bulge in the central tympanic membrane.
- For optimal results, the head of the Spandrel II should remain as large as possible.
- The stability of the level of the tympanic membrane is critical in the neomalleus reconstruction. Staging is therefore essential.
- The prosthesis is applied to the neomalleus to confirm the proper length for a 0.5–mm protrusion in the vestibule. This requires repositioning of the tympanomeatal flap.
- In a thick drum, a one-stage neomalleus ossiculoplasty is possible. The pouch is made with microtympanoplasty scissors. Care should be taken to accurately form the pouch to assure most-stable fixation for proper adaptation of the stapedotomy prosthesis.
- The space available for stapedotomy in neomalleus procedures is more limited than that in stapedotomy for otosclerosis. Even the smallest movements of the tympanomeatal flap may dislocate the prosthesis.

Chapter 4
Special Applications with Tympanoplasty

1. Transcanal Myringotomy with Ventilating Tube

Transcanal myringotomy with ventilating tube (Grommet) is used when chronic serous otitis media is accompanied by a conductive hearing loss of 30 dB or more. *Temporary* ventilating tubes are used first. If a repeated temporary ventilation tube fails, a *permanent* ventilating tube is introduced. A *myringotomy* alone is used as symptomatic treatment in: acute suppurative otitis media, barotrauma, and as an adjunct procedure in acute mastoiditis. Myringotomy with a ventilating tube is rarely used in conjunction with tympanoplasty. In the latter case, a transmastoid drain is preferred (see Fig. **56**, p. 106). This enables cleaning the middle ear of secretions and securing postoperative ventilation.

1.1 Temporary Ventilating Tube (Grommet)

Surgical Technique

This procedure is performed under general anesthesia for children and local anesthesia for adults. Local anesthesia is provided with Gingicain spray (2% tetracaine) applied over the tympanic membrane 5 minutes prior to myringotomy.

Surgical Highlights

- Local anesthesia (adults), general anesthesia (children)
- Transcanal approach through ear speculum
- Radial myringotomy in anteroinferior quadrant of the tympanic membrane
- Transportation of the Grommet with 1.5-mm, 45° hook
- Introduction of inner flange of the Grommet through the myringotomy opening with a 1.5-mm, 45° hook.

Surgical Steps

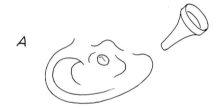

Fig. 64 A

Ear speculum

The ear speculum is introduced and kept in place with the left hand.

Fig. 64 B

Myringotomy

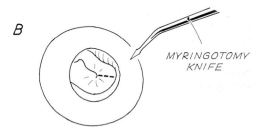

The myringotomy is performed with a myringotomy knife in the anteroinferior quadrant of the drum. A radial incision is preferred to a circumferential to avoid infolding of the incision's margins and subsequent formation of cholesteatoma (see also Fig. **7 B**). The length of the incision should match the diameter of the inner flange of the Grommet. The incision should avoid the tympanic annulus to prevent early extrusion. In the presence of a retracted drum, the myringotomy should be made within the deepest available space in the hypotympanum.

Fig. 64 C

Transportation of ventilating tube

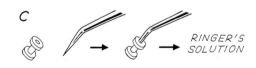

Many kinds and shapes of ventilating tubes are available. Our preference are "homemade" polyethylene tubes of various size (PE 50, PE 60). The flanges of the tubes are created by placing the cut end of the tubes over a hot metal surface. The tubes are sterilized prior to use. The tube is picked up using a 45°, 1.5-mm hook and placed in Ringer's solution. A wet ventilating tube is less prone to slide away along the tympanic membrane during placement.

Fig. 64 D

Transportation of ventilating tube (cont.)

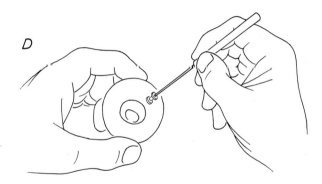

The ear speculum is kept in position with the left hand, and the ventilating tube is introduced into the external auditory canal with the right hand.

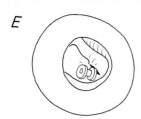

Fig. **64 E**

Ventilating tube on tympanic membrane

The tube is placed on the tympanic membrane close to the myringotomy opening.

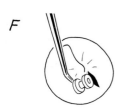

Fig. **64 F**

Introduction of ventilating tube

The 1.5-mm, 45° hook is used to place the inner flange of the tube over the myringotomy incision.

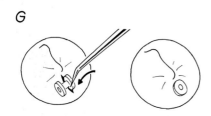

Fig. **64 G**

Introduction of ventilating tube (cont.)

The inner flange of the tube is rotated into the tympanic cavity using the 1.5-mm, 45° hook.

1.2 Permanent Ventilating T-Tube (Grommet)

Surgical Technique

For permanent ventilation, our preference is a Goode T-Grommet, Xomed Product No. 40812. This tube remains in place up to 3 years. After this, a chronic perforation of the tympanic membrane may result in 10% of the cases.

Surgical Highlights

- Local anesthesia (adults), general anesthesia (children)
- Modification of T tube
- Introduction of T tube with small alligator forceps

Surgical Steps

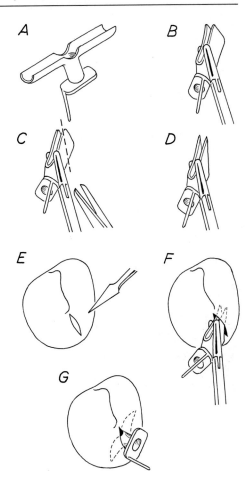

Fig. **65** Permanent Ventilating T-Tube

A: Goode T-Grommet Silicon ventilating tube

B: The flanges of the tube are grasped with a straight alligator forceps

C: Trimming the flanges of the T-Grommet

D: Modified T-Grommet ready for introduction

E: Myringotomy in the anteroinferior quadrant of the drum

F: The flanges of the T-ventilating tube are grasped with small alligator forceps and inserted through the myringotomy incision

G: Final position of T-ventilating tube

2. Temporary Round Window Electrode

Surgical Technique

A temporary round window electrode is used to test whether a patient with bilateral deafness is suitable for a cochlear implant.

Surgical Highlights

- Local anesthesia
- Endaural approach
- Limited tympanomeatal flap
- Notch for electrode drilled in posterior canal wall below the chorda tympani
- Fixation of electrode on the round window membrane and in the notch of the external auditory canal
- Threading of electrode through meatal skin in the postauricular region

Surgical Steps

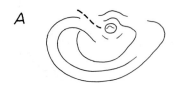

A

Fig. 66 A

Endaural skin incision

The helicotragal incision is carried out as for stapedotomy.

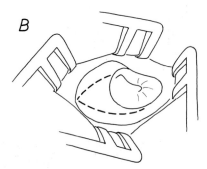

B

Fig. 66 B

Tympanomeatal flap

The posterior limbs of the tympanomeatal flap are carried out more caudal than for stapes surgery.

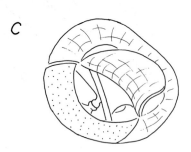

C

Fig. 66 C

Exposure of round window

The tympanomeatal flap is elevated and the chorda tympani dissected free. The round window niche is exposed below the chorda.

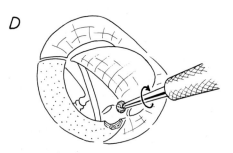

D

Fig. 66 D

Electrode notch drilled in posterior canal wall

A notch for fixation of the electrode is drilled with a diamond burr in the posterior canal wall. The direction of rotation of the burr is away from the chorda tympani.

Fig. 66 E

Insertion and fixation of electrode

The ball end of the insulated platinum iridium electrode is applied on the round window membrane. If necessary, the electrode is fixed in the notch of the posterior canal wall with a drop of Histoacryl glue or with Ionocement (see instrumentation).

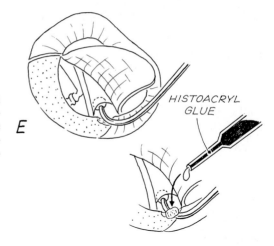

Fig. 66 F

Threading of electrode through posterior canal wall

The posterior end of a large injection needle is cut away with strong scissors to allow passage of the electrode. The injection needle is introduced from the retroauricular skin into the lumen of the external auditory canal. The lateral end of the electrode is passed through the needle and brought out behind the pinna.

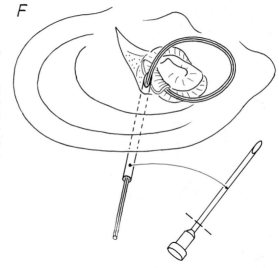

Fig. 66 G

Retroauricular fixation of the round window electrode

Steristrips are used to fix the electrode in the retroauricular region. The electrode remains in place for 2 days. After testing, the electrode is removed by pulling it through the skin. Care must be taken to use a very small amount of glue to fix the electrode to the notch in the posterior canal wall to avoid pain when removing it.

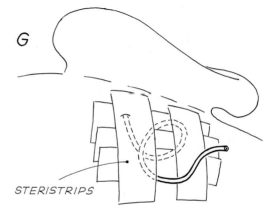

3. Canalplasty for Exostosis

Surgical Technique

Indication. Retention of cerumen and keratin in the external canal with recurrent episodes of external otitis.

Surgical Principle. Removal of external canal exostoses requires complete elimination of overhanging bone lateral to the tympanic annulus. The shape of the bony external canal should be an inverted, truncated cone. The meatal skin flaps should be kept intact to promote rapid reepithelization of the enlarged canal. To keep the canal skin intact, the posterior bony overhang should be removed first, the anterior second.

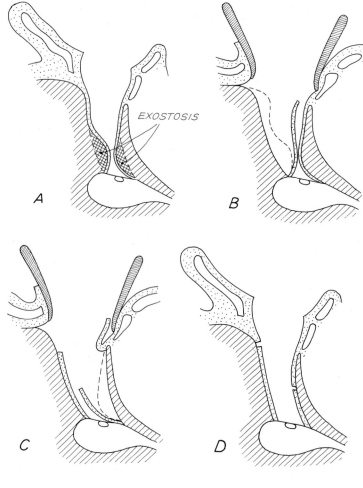

Fig. **67**

Principles of canalplasty for exostosis

A: Preoperative view showing the narrowing of the canal due to the exostosis.

B: Elevation of posterior meatal skin flap and removal of posterior exostosis.

C: Elevation of anterior meatal skin flap and removal of anterior exostosis.

D: Completed canalplasty.

Surgical Highlights

- Endaural approach
- Posterior and anterior meatal skin flaps
- Total removal of bony overhangs lateral to tympanic annulus
- Replacement of preserved meatal skin flaps

Surgical Steps

Fig. 68 A

Skin incision

Helicotragal incision as for stapedotomy.

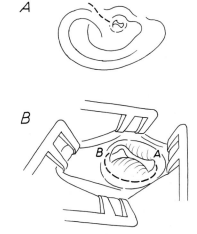

Fig. 68 B

Posterior meatal incision

The entrance of the external auditory canal is enlarged with two endaural retractors. A posterior semicircumferential incision (A–B) is carried out along the lateral edge of the exostotic bone.

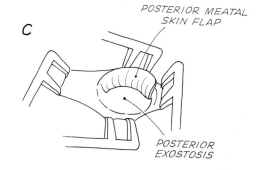

Fig. 68 C

Elevation of posterior meatal flap

The skin is elevated over the posterior exostotic bone. Vertical incisions along the bony canal wall are carried out at 12 o'clock and 6 o'clock using tympanoplasty microscissors.

POSTERIOR MEATAL
SKIN FLAP

POSTERIOR
EXOSTOSIS

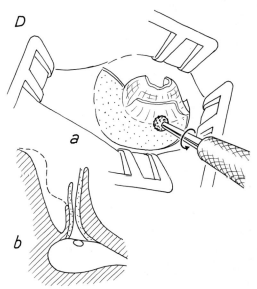

Fig. 68 D

Removal of posterior exostosis

a: A diamond burr is used to remove the excess of bone along the posterior canal wall. The rotation of the burr is away from the elevated meatal skin. Preservation of the canal skin is essential to promote rapid postoperative epithelization

b: A thin layer of bone covering the elevated skin is left behind while drilling away the excess of bone along the posterior canal wall to protect the skin.

E

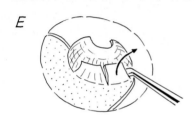

Fig. **68 E**

Removal of posterior exostosis (cont.)

When the tympanic annulus is reached, the egg-shell of bone protecting the meatal skin is broken off with the "universal" microraspatory.

ANTERIOR   POSTERIOR
EXOSTOSIS   MEATAL
              SKIN FLAP

F

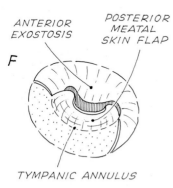

Fig. **68 F**

Removal of posterior exostosis (cont.)

Surgical site following complete removal of the posterior exostosis, showing the tympanic annulus and the intact meatal skin.

TYMPANIC ANNULUS

G

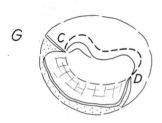

Fig. **68 G**

Anterior meatal incision

An anterior semicircumferential incision is carried out along the lateral margin of the anterior exostosis (C–D).

H

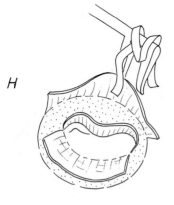

Fig. **68 H**

Elevation of lateral meatal skin

The skin covering the anterior entrance of the external canal is elevated and retracted from the lumen with an aluminium strip anchored to the retroauricular retractor (see also Fig. **87**, p. 169).

Fig. 68 I

Removal of anterior exostosis

a: The anterior excess of bone is removed with a diamond drill. The rotation of the burr is always away from the meatal skin (*a*).

b: A thin layer of bone is left back to protect the skin flap until the anterior tympanic annulus is reached (*b*). Care should be taken to avoid breaking into the temporomandibular joint with the burr. Drilling should be discontinued if a pink–gray discoloration is noted through the bone under irrigation.

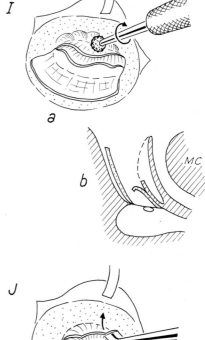

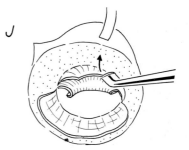

Fig. 68 J

Removal of anterior exostosis (cont.)

The last eggshell of bone protecting the meatal skin is removed with the "universal" microraspatory, remaining lateral to the tympanic annulus.

Fig. 68 K

Extent of bone removal in canalplasty

Correct widening of the external auditory canal implies elimination of all overhanging bone lateral to the tympanic annulus. Failure to open the tympanomeatal angle at the level of the annulus results in the accumulation of keratin with recurrence of exostosis.

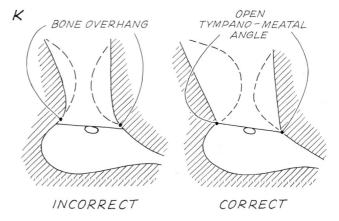

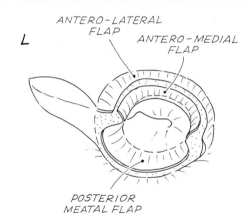

L

ANTERO-LATERAL FLAP

ANTERO-MEDIAL FLAP

POSTERIOR MEATAL FLAP

Fig. **68 L**

Final positioning of meatal skin flaps

The shape of the external auditory canal is that of an inverted truncated cone. The meatal skin flaps are repositioned. The original meatal skin completely covers the enlarged lumen of the canal. Reepithelization occurs within 3 to 4 weeks.

4. Canalplasty for Otitis Externa Obliterans

Surgical Technique

Indication. Obliteration of the external auditory canal lumen following chronic external otitis defeating medical treatment. The hearing loss should be 20 dB or more.

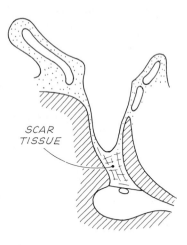

SCAR TISSUE

Fig. **69**

Schematic representation of otitis externa obliterans

The narrow bony lumen of the external auditory canal is obliterated by scar tissue. The fibrous layer of the tympanic membrane is intact. The intraluminal scar tissue is covered by skin.

Surgical Highlights

- Local anesthesia
- Endaural approach
- Removal of obliterative scar, keeping the fibrous layer of the tympanic membrane intact

- Elimination of bone overhangs lateral to the tympanic annulus
- Skin grafting of the fibrous tympanic membrane and bony external canal

Surgical Steps

Fig. 70 A

Endaural Incision

Helicotragal skin incision as for stapedotomy.

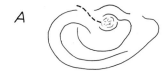

Fig. 70 B

Meatal skin flap

Semicircumferential incision (*A–B*) at the posterior entrance of the external auditory canal.

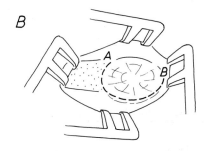

Fig. 70 C

Elevation of lateral canal skin

The skin covering the obliterative scar is elevated out of the meatus and retracted anteriorly with the endaural retractors.

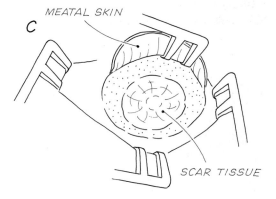

Fig. 70 D

Removal of obliterative scar

The "universal" microraspatory is used to elevate the scar tissue occluding the bony canal. The medial plane of cleavage is along the tympanic annulus and inferior pars tensa. Identification of the correct plane of cleavage allows preservation of the fibrous pars tensa and avoids laceration of the Shrapnell membrane.

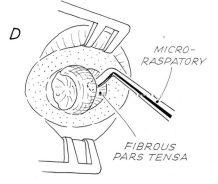

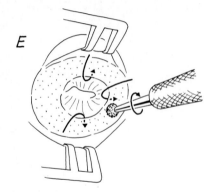

Fig. **70 E**

Canalplasty

The bony overhang of the canal wall is removed with a diamond burr until the complete tympanic annulus can be seen with one position of the microscope.

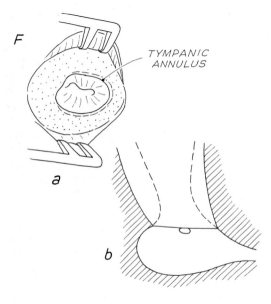

TYMPANIC
ANNULUS

Fig. **70 F**

Completed canalplasty (cont.)

a: The tympanic annulus is completely exposed.

b: There is no bony overhang *(dotted line)* lateral to the annulus.

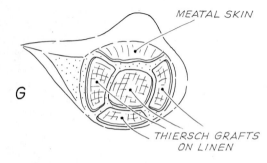

MEATAL SKIN

THIERSCH GRAFTS
ON LINEN

Fig. **70 G**

Skin grafting of external auditory canal

The original meatal skin covers only a limited anterior area of the canal wall. Split-thickness skin grafts (Thiersch) are obtained from the inner surface of the opposite upper arm of the patient. They are applied with their keratin side on linen (see Fig. 72 K, p. 138) over the fibrous tympanic membrane and the bare bony canal walls.

5. Congenital Aural Atresia

Definition

Congenital aural atresia may vary from *mild* (hypoplastic external canal with normal tympanic cavity) to *severe* (complete absence of external canal with very small or missing tympanic cavity). The surgical techniques described on the following pages relate to the Altmann type II congenital atresia (absent external auditory canal, ossicular malformation and bony atresia plate lateral to the tympanic cavity).

Indications for Surgery

a) *Bilateral atresia.* Functional surgery in bilateral atresia is performed at the age of 5–6 years (before the beginning of primary school). Only one side is operated upon. Surgery of the second ear is carried out only after puberty, when the patient can give his or her own consent.
b) *Unilateral atresia.* Unilateral atretic ears are operated on only after puberty, when the patient can make his or her own decision for or against surgery.
c) *Plastic reconstruction of the malformed auricle.* It is advisable to perform plastic reconstruction of the malformed auricle with cooperation between the plastic and otologic surgeons. The possibility of a bone-anchored epithetic prosthesis or of leaving the malformed ear as it is until the patient can decide on his or her own is also discussed with the parents.

Prerequisites for Surgery

The prerequisites for successful functional surgery of an atretic ear are:

– Sufficient pneumatization of the middle ear
– Presence of identifiable ossicular remnants on high-resolution CT scans
– Adequate cochlear function
– Sufficient cooperation of patients and parents

Anatomy of the Congenital Atretic Ear

Atresia of the external auditory canal is caused by a malformation of the tympanic bone, leading to the underdevelopment of the cavum tympani below the chorda. The malleus handle is usually fused to the malformed tympanic bone (atresia plate). The upper half of the middle ear cavity, particularly the epitympanum, is normally formed. The inferior half of the mastoid process is malformed and may lead to an abnormal position of the fallopian canal (Fig. **71**). Surgical rehabilitation of the atretic ear should take into consideration that the abnormality is mostly confined to the inferior tympanic cavity. Therefore, the initial approach *should be* from superior through the attic rather than from posterior through the mastoid. The ossicles are best identified in the epitympanic space where they are least affected by the malformation. The "new" tympanic cavity should be centered at the level of the lateral process of the malleus and *not*—as in a normal ear—at the umbo. The malformed ossicles *should not* be sacrificed for restoration of hearing. The malformed incus and stapes are usually mobile. The malleus becomes mobile when the malformed handle is separated from the atresia plate. The facial nerve is best identified above the oval window. EMG monitoring of facial function (NIM-2*) is mandatory. One must realize that the newly formed external auditory canal has a different position than in a normal ear because the epitympanum is included in the new tympanic cavity. Many textbooks convey the wrong idea that in congenital atresia, reconstruction of a "normal" external auditory canal and of a normal middle ear cavity are possible.

---

* Xomed-Treace

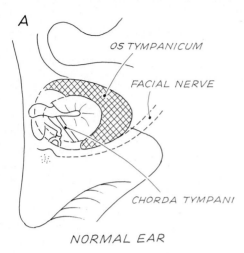

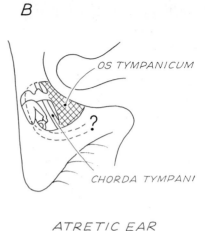

Fig. 71

Anatomy of the normal and atretic ear

A: Normal tympanic bone.

B: Malformed tympanic bone with hypoplastic inferior tympanic space and mastoid. The tympanic segment of the facial nerve is usually in the normal position above the oval window niche. On the other hand, the mastoid segment can take a variable course in the malformed mastoid.

5.1 Surgery for Aural Atresia

Surgical Technique

The following surgical steps describe a case of tympanoplasty without reconstruction of the auricle (for the latter, see p. 140).

Surgical Highlights

- General anesthesia
- Z-plasty for posterior transposition of the auricular remnant
- Epitympanotomy for identification of malleus and incus
- Removal of atresia plate and canalplasty
- Mobilization of ossicular chain by separation of malleus handle from atresia plate
- Inclusion of the epitympanum in the "new" tympanic cavity
- Overlay grafting of tympanic membrane with temporalis fascia
- Skin grafting of overlaid fascia and new bony external canal
- Anchoring of skin flap to the entrance of the new external auditory canal.

Surgical Steps

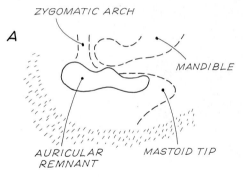

Fig. 72 A

Surgical site in atretic ear

The malformed tympanic bone and root of zygoma place the mastoid in direct contact with the temporomandibular joint.

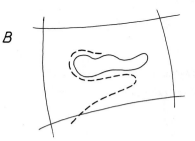

Fig. 72 B

Skin incision for Z-plasty

The skin incision for the Z-plasty is designed to move the upper auricular remnant posteriorly.

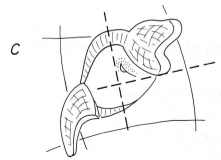

Fig. 72 C

Locating the epitympanum (attic)

The position of the attic is obtained by drawing two perpendicular lines along the posterior and superior margins of the temporomandibular fossa. The attic lies along the superior, horizontal line and anterior to the crossing point of both lines.

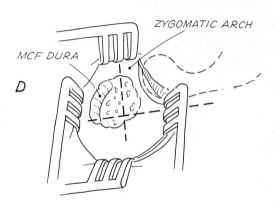

Fig. 72 D

Epitympanotomy

Drilling begins with exposure of the middle cranial fossa dura leaving enough bone for its protection.

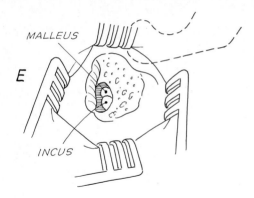

E

MALLEUS

INCUS

Fig. **72 E**

Exposure of malleus and incus

Drilling along the middle cranial fossa dura leads to the pneumatic spaces surrounding the malleus head and the incus body at the depth of 1 cm.

Fig. **72 F**

Removal of the atresia plate and formation of a new bony canal

The atretic tympanic bone is removed, forming the new external auditory canal. A shell of anterior bone is left over the temporomandibular joint to avoid prolapse of soft tissues into the lumen of the new canal. Note that the malformed malleus handle is incorporated with the atresia plate below the chorda tympani. The chorda tympani indicates the position of the mastoid segment of the facial nerve. The use of facial nerve monitoring (NIM-2) is mandatory when drilling posterior to the chorda tympani. Care should be taken to widen the new canal as much as possible around the malleus handle. A small bridge of bone is preserved at the tip of the malformed malleus to insure its fixation until completion of the canalplasty.

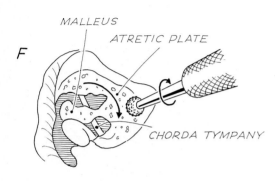

F

MALLEUS

ATRETIC PLATE

CHORDA TYMPANY

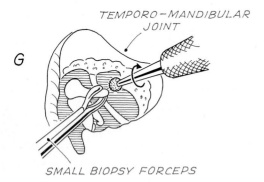

G

TEMPORO-MANDIBULAR JOINT

SMALL BIOPSY FORCEPS

Fig. **72 G**

Mobilization of the ossicular chain

After the canalplasty is completed, the malleus is stabilized with a small biopsy forceps (left hand) while the last bridge of bone fixing it to the atresia plate is removed with a diamond drill (right hand). This maneuver restores the normal mobility of the malformed ossicular chain.

Fig. 72 H

Identification of facial nerve and formation of a new tympanic sulcus

The tympanic segment of the facial nerve is identified above the oval window. The malformed long process of the incus has a steeper angle than in normal ears. The stapes arch may be malformed but is usually mobile. A *new tympanic sulcus* is drilled from the middle cranial fossa dura (anterosuperiorly) to the short process of the incus (posteriorly). The new tympanic cavity is centered on the incudomallear joint.

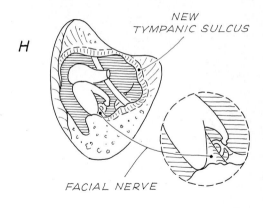

Fig. 72 I

Harvesting of the temporalis fascia

The new external canal is completed. A piece of fascia is obtained from the lateral surface of the temporalis muscle *(broken line)*.

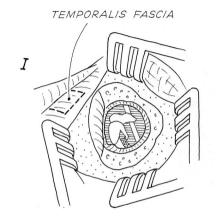

Fig. 72 J

Anchoring sutures for the skin flaps

Anchoring the skin flaps to the bone is very important to avoid secondary stenosis of the new external canal. For this purpose, several holes are created with a diamond burr (*A*) along the lateral edge of the new canal. Care should be taken to avoid injuring the middle fossa dura when drilling the superior holes. 4–0 Vicryl sutures are passed with watchmaker forceps through the anchoring holes (*B*). These sutures are used to secure the skin flaps to the bone at the end of the procedure.

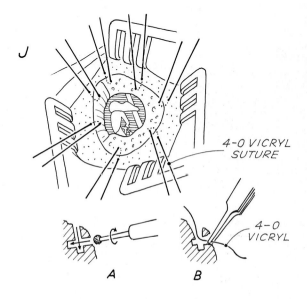

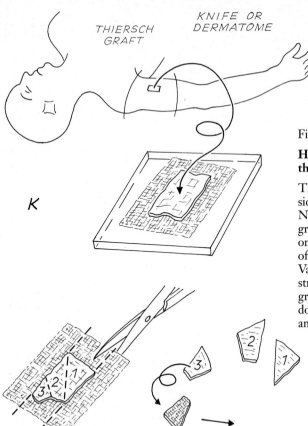

Fig. **72 K**

Harvesting and preparation of split-thickness skin grafts (Thiersch)

Thiersch grafts are obtained from the inner side of the upper arm of the patient with a No. 20 blade or with a dermatome. The grafts are placed with their keratin surface on a piece of linen covered with a thin layer of Vaseline. The skin graft attached to the Vaseline linen is cut in smaller pieces using straight scissors. The smaller Thiersch grafts will be turned with their dermal side downward to cover the temporalis fascia and the bony external canal.

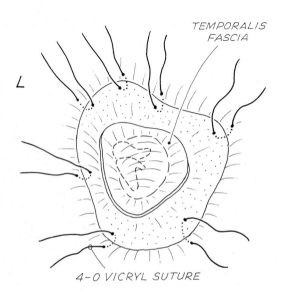

Fig. **72 L**

Overlay graft

The resected temporalis fascia is placed over a glass board, and excess muscle and fat are removed with a knife (see Fig. 14 F, p. 28). The fresh fascia is then used as an overlay graft to cover the ossicles and the new tympanic sulcus.

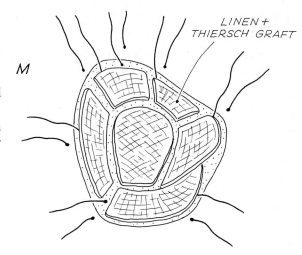

LINEN +
THIERSCH GRAFT

M

Fig. 72 M

Skin grafting of fascial graft and canal wall

Various Thiersch grafts on Vaseline linen are used to cover the overlaid temporalis fascia and the bony external canal.

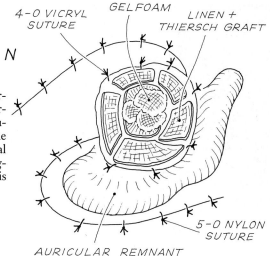

4-0 VICRYL SUTURE

GELFOAM

LINEN + THIERSCH GRAFT

N

5-0 NYLON SUTURE

AURICULAR REMNANT

Fig. 72 N

Wound closure and packing

The flaps of the Z-plasty are transposed. The margins of the skin flaps are anchored to the lateral surface of the external canal with the 4–0 Vicryl sutures threaded through the holes drilled in the bone (see Fig. 72 J). The lumen of the external auditory canal is packed with Gelfoam impregnated with Otosporin. The remaining wound is closed with 5–0 nylon sutures.

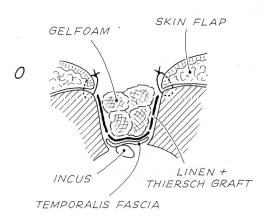

GELFOAM

SKIN FLAP

O

INCUS

LINEN + THIERSCH GRAFT

TEMPORALIS FASCIA

Fig. 72 O

Wound closure and packing (cont.)

Schematic representation of the skin margins anchored to the entrance of the external canal. The Gelfoam pledgets keep the fascia and the Thiersch grafts in contact with the mobilized ossicles and the bony wall of the external canal.

5.2 Surgery for Aural Atresia in Combination with Plastic Reconstruction of the External Canal

Plastic reconstruction of the auricle in combination with correction of conductive hearing loss is gaining increased acceptance throughout the world. The reconstruction of the auricle is performed first. Canalplasty and tympanoplasty are carried out in an intermediate stage when the main part of the reconstructed auricle is in place.

Surgical Technique

A retroauricular incision may be used if repositioning of the reconstructed auricle is needed. The following surgical steps relate to the situation of an appropriate position of the external ear.

Surgical Highlights

- General anesthesia
- Endaural skin incision
- Epitympanotomy
- Canalplasty
- Mobilization of ossicular chain
- Overlay grafting with temporalis fascia
- Skin grafting of overlaid fascia and external auditory canal
- Skin margins secured to the bony entrance of the external canal by anchoring sutures

Surgical Steps

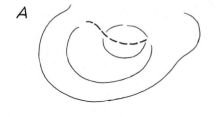

Fig. **73 A**

Endaural skin incision

Helicotragal incision as for stapedotomy at the level of the estimated new opening of the external auditory canal.

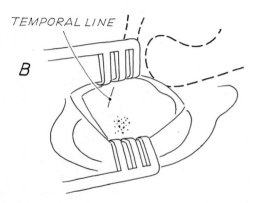

Fig. **73 B**

Locating the epitympanum

The estimated position of the epitympanum is below the temporal line and posterior to the temporomandibular joint (see also Fig. 72 C, p.135).

Fig. **73 C**

Epitympanotomy and identification of the ossicles

The attic is open. The head of the malleus and the body of the incus are exposed by drilling away the bone along the middle fossa dura.

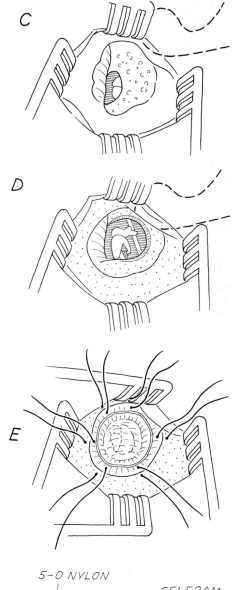

Fig. **73 D**

Canalplasty and mobilization of the ossicular chain

The atresia plate is drilled away, forming a new external auditory canal. The malleus handle is mobilized as demonstrated in Figs. 72 F and G, p. 136. A new tympanic sulcus is formed around the mobilized ossicle as shown in Fig. 72 H, p. 137.

Fig. **73 E**

Anchoring sutures for skin margins

Holes are drilled through the lateral entrance of the bony auditory canal (see also Fig. 72 J). 4–0 Vicryl sutures are placed through the holes to anchor the skin margins. A free temporalis fascia graft is used as an overlay to cover the mobilized ossicles and the new tympanic sulcus.

Fig. **73 F**

Anchoring of skin margins

Thiersch grafts mounted on linen are used to cover the overlaid fascia and the bony wall of the external canal. The skin margins are anchored to the entrance of the canal using 4–0 Vicryl sutures. The endaural incision is closed with 5–0 nylon sutures.

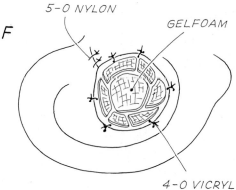

5–0 NYLON

GELFOAM

4–0 VICRYL

5.3 Results of Congenital Atretic Ear Correction

Surgery for the atretic ear is difficult because the middle ear and facial nerve anatomy are distorted. Formation of a wide, self-cleaning external auditory canal with avoidance of subsequent stenosis and successful reconstruction of the sound-conductive mechanism are not easy to achieve. The results obtained using the techniques described in the preceding section demonstrate the problems involved in the management of the atretic ear.

Table **12** shows the hearing results of 32 patients who underwent surgery consecutively because of severe ear atresia. Fifteen patients underwent a traditional mastoidectomy; 17 patients underwent the anterior epitympanotomy approach. All patients have been followed up for at least 3 years postoperatively. The improvements in air conduction and in the residual air–bone gap were measured for the speech frequencies (500, 1000, and 2000 Hz). The anterior atticotomy gave superior results to the mastoidectomy. Forty-one percent of the patients with the anterior (atticotomy) approach closed the air–bone gap within 0–30 dB. However, even with the atticotomy approach, an equal number (41%) of patients presented a residual air–bone gap of more than 40 dB 5 years postoperatively. This means that obtaining normal hearing on a long-term basis still remains an illusory goal in 59% of the patients with atretic ears. However, patients with "unsuccessful" hearing results may still benefit from the possibility of wearing a hearing aid.

The complications of surgery of the atretic ear are shown in Table **13**. No postoperative facial paralysis or weakness was noted in any patient who had undergone surgery. The incidence of otorrhea and restenosis of the external canal was reduced to one-fifth and one-third, respectively with the anterior (atticotomy) approach. Stent material for the external canal was not used because it was found to stimulate rather than to prevent cicatricial conditions*.

---

* Mattox DE, Fisch U. Otolaryngol Head Neck Surg 1986; 94: 574–577.

Table **12** Hearing results in surgical correction of severe aural atresia (n = 32, 5-year follow-up)

Improvement of air conduction (dB)	Mastoidectomy		Atticotomy	
	n	(%)	n	(%)
> 40	–	–	3/17	(18)
> 31	1/15	(7)	8/17	(47)
≤ 30	14/15	(93)	9/17	(53)
Residual air–bone gap (dB)				
0–10	–	(–)	–	(–)
0–20	1/15	(7)	4/17	(24)
0–30	1/15	(7)	7/17	(41)
0–40	3/15	(20)	10/17	(59)
40	12/15	(80)	7/17	(41)

Table **13** Complications in surgical correction of congenital atresia (n = 32, 5-year follow-up)

Approach	Otorrhea		External canal stenosis	
	n	(%)	n	(%)
Mastoidectomy	5/15	(33)	5/15	(33)
Atticotomy	1/17	(6)	2/17	(12)

6. Rules and Hints

- Facial nerve monitoring is mandatory in surgery of an atretic ear.
- Suturing skin flaps to bone prevents stenosis of the new external canal.
- Preserve the ossicular tissues whenever possible.
- It is necessary to open the anterior external canal widely without violating the temporomandibular joint.
- Avoid opening the mastoid cells when forming the new external canal.
- Remove the atresia plate surrounding the malformed malleus handle as much as possible to avoid later refixation.
- The mobilization of the malleus from the atresia plate may cause trauma to the inner ear.
- Anchoring the skin flaps to bone avoids the need for stenting the external canal.
- Leave the split-thickness skin grafts with the initial packing for 2 weeks.

- Be certain to remove all pieces of Vaseline linen placed for fixation of the split-thickness graft in the canal after 2 weeks to avoid foreign body reaction.
- Use diamond burrs rather than cutting burrs when working close to the temporomandibular joint.
- Keep the meatal skin flaps intact when enlarging a stenotic canal because otherwise reepithelization may be severely retarded and the possibility of restenosis increased.
- Long-standing ventilating tubes carry an increased risk of permanent perforation.
- Operated atretic or stenotic canals require prolonged débridement until healing is complete.
- Any chronic secretion in the operated external canal carries the risk of restenosis and conductive hearing loss.

Chapter 5
Mastoidectomy

General Considerations

1. Definitions

Disease involving the middle ear can extend to the mastoid and require surgical procedures involving this bone. Surgery limited to the mastoid is defined as *cortical* or *simple mastoidectomy*. A cortical mastoidectomy is mainly carried out in acute mastoiditis to drain infected mastoid air cells in association with myringotomy and introduction of a ventilating tube. Acute viral mastoiditis with inner ear involvement (vertigo and sensorineural hearing loss) requires mastoidectomy combined with epitympanectomy and posterior tympanotomy. This is necessary to achieve adequate drainage of the round and oval window niche, preventing permanent inner ear damage.

In this chapter, mastoidectomy is mainly discussed in association with the treatment of middle ear disease (tympanomastoidectomy). The term *intact canal wall* or *closed cavity tympanomastoidectomy* is used when the posterosuperior canal wall is preserved. The term *canal wall down* or *open cavity tympanomastoidectomy* implies removal of the posterosuperior canal wall. The most common indication for a tympanomastoidectomy is chronic otitis media complicated by a cholesteatoma.

2. Cholesteatoma

Cholesteatoma is defined as the presence of keratinizing squamous epithelium within the middle ear or in other pneumatized areas of the temporal bone.

3. Classification of Cholesteatoma

The cholesteatoma may be classified as

– **Congenital**
– **Primary acquired**
– **Secondary acquired**

---

* For management of congenital cholesteatoma see Fisch U, Mattox DE. Microsurgery of the Skull Base. Stuttgart: Georg Thieme Verlag, 1988.

a) Congenital Cholesteatoma*

Congenital cholesteatoma is a developmental defect consisting of a cystic epidermoid growth arising from rests of keratinizing squamous epithelium present before birth. The patients have no history of ear disease and a normally pneumatized mastoid.

b) Acquired Cholesteatoma

Acquired cholesteatoma occurs after birth and is caused by invasion of the middle ear cleft by keratinizing squamous epithelium originating from the lining of the external auditory canal or from the tympanic membrane (Table **14**). Patients with acquired cholesteatoma usually present with a history of recurrent ear disease and with a reduced pneumatization of the mastoid. According to the condition of the tympanic membrane, acquired cholesteatoma can be divided into *primary* and *secondary*. *Primary acquired cholesteatomas* develop behind an intact tympanic membrane. *Secondary acquired cholesteatomas* grow in the middle ear through a mostly marginal perforation of the tympanic membrane.

Acquired cholesteatomas most commonly originate from a large posterosuperior perforation or from a small superior attic perforation. According to a study performed under F. R. Nager in the ENT Department, University Hospital, Zürich, Switzerland, before the antibiotic era, intracranial compli-

cations occurred in only 1.7% of cholesteatomas with extensive posterosuperior drum defects and in 6% of the cases with small attic perforations. Out of 763 cases of cholesteatomatous otitis media reviewed in 1934 by Nager, 631 cases presented with a large posterosuperior perforation. The middle ear suppuration started as a necrotizing otitis media of infancy in 35% of the cases. This arose in the course of scarlet fever, measles, diphtheria, tuberculosis, or influenza. In the remaining 65% of cholesteatomas with large perforations, no such history could be obtained. Since the middle ear infection dated from early childhood in the majority of cases, it was assumed that cholesteatomas with large perforations also begin in infancy as a necrotizing otitis media of unknown etiology.

Only 20% of the 132 cases with a small attic perforation presented with a history of otitis media in early childhood. In none of the cases could the ENT specialist observe the appearance of a small upper marginal perforation in the course of the acute otitis media. At the onset, the disease was usually

Table **14**   Chain of events in the development of acquired cholesteatoma

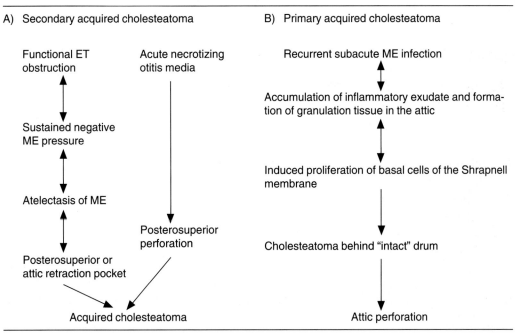

symptomless and without an obvious association of a middle ear infection. A small perforation was often discovered accidentally in the course of a routine examination.

There is no doubt today that in the presence of large posterosuperior perforations, as first described by Habermann in 1889 (Fig. **74**), meatal epithelium grows inward through the perforation and, once in the middle ear, stimulates the production of a cholesteatoma (immigration theory). On the other hand, controversy still exists concerning the pathogenesis of the attic cholesteatomas. In 1958 L. Rüedi carried out an extensive histological and experimental study on the pathogenesis of cholesteatoma. He has shown that the pathogenesis of primary and secondary acquired attic cholesteatomas can best be explained on the basis of the immigration theory. Lange first put forward the opinion that a prolonged inflammatory stimulus may induce the proliferation of the basal cells in the epidermis of the Shrapnell membrane (Fig. **74**). Rüedi opened the aural bulla in guinea pigs and introduced a mixture of talc and fibrin underneath the internal surface of the intact tympanic membrane. This caused a mild foreign body reaction, and in several animals, granulation tissue developed between the drum and internal wall of the middle ear. Active ingrowth of the epidermis from the intact tympanic membrane into the newly formed granulation tissue was found to occur after 15–20 days. Invading colonies

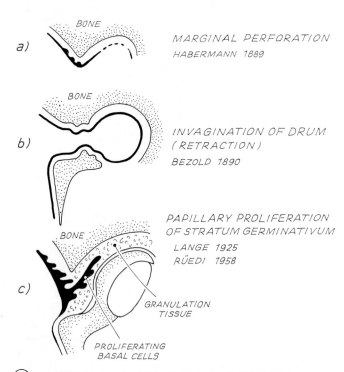

PATHOGENESIS OF ACQUIRED CHOLESTEATOMA

(1) INGROWTH OF SQUAMOUS EPITHELIUM

a) BONE

MARGINAL PERFORATION
HABERMANN 1889

b) BONE

INVAGINATION OF DRUM
(RETRACTION)
BEZOLD 1890

c) BONE

PAPILLARY PROLIFERATION
OF STRATUM GERMINATIVUM
LANGE 1925
RÜEDI 1958

GRANULATION
TISSUE

PROLIFERATING
BASAL CELLS

(2) METAPLASIA OF MIDDLE EAR MUCOSA
ULRICH 1917
SADÉ 1977

Fig. **74**

Pathogenesis of acquired cholesteatoma

of basal cells divided into branches, and the desquamated stratified squamous epithelium formed typical cholesteatomatous masses. The clinical and histological study of normal and pathological animal experiments led Rüedi to the conclusion that, as a rule, all types of cholesteatoma of the middle ear develop by immigration of stratified squamous epithelium from the epidermis of the external auditory meatus or the tympanic membrane. Within the middle ear cavities, the active growth of the matrix is enhanced by submucous connective tissue filling the incompletely pneumatized attic and epitympanic cells. A search for evidence of embryonic cell rests or areas of metaplasia in the mucosa of the middle ear proved fruitless in 124 temporal bones obtained from patients with cholesteatoma, acute otitis media, and from normal young children examined histologically by serial section. While the occurrence of such cell rests or metaplasia is possible (Fig. 74), it is at best very rare, whereas cholesteatomas are commonly encountered.

The lesson to be learned from Rüedi's investigations is that any inflammatory reaction occurring in the pneumatic space of the attic may potentially induce a cholesteatoma. This is why we consider epitympanectomy (see p. 96) a must in the presence of chronic attic disease.

Secondary acquired cholesteatomas are divided according to their origin into the following types.

– *Iatrogenic* (keratinizing epithelium introduced in the middle ear cavity by a surgical procedure)

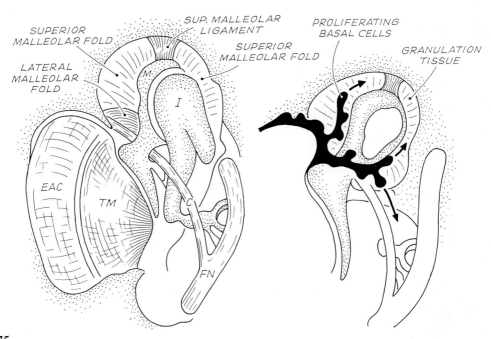

Fig. 75

Routes of invasion of primary acquired cholesteatoma of the attic

A primary acquired cholesteatoma may occur under an apparently intact tympanic membrane when the membrana limitans of the epithelium of the Shrapnell membrane is injured by a chronic infection with granulation tissue in the attic. The proliferating basal cells of the Shrapnell membrane penetrate into the granulation tissue through a hole of the membrana limitans without visible external perforation. The primary cholesteatoma differs from the congenital cholesteatoma because it is accompanied by a history of middle ear infection in a (mostly) sclerotic mastoid.

– *Residual* (rest of keratinizing epithelium remaining after a surgical procedure)
– *Recurrent* (new secondary acquired cholesteatoma appearing following complete removal of a previous one)
– *Retention cholesteatoma* (accumulation of keratin in an insufficiently exteriorized cavity). This latter type of cholesteatoma is not strictly confined to the middle ear (mucosal lined cavity) but can also develop within the insufficiently enlarged external auditory canal.

ACQUIRED CHOLESTEATOMA OF THE ATTIC

LATERAL ROUTE ⟶

MEDIAL ROUTE ╍╍╍⟶

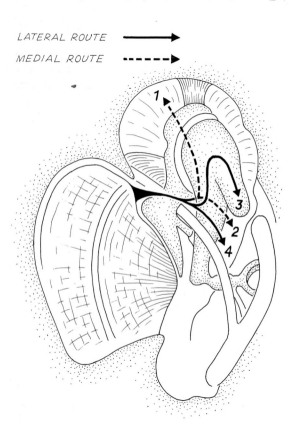

Fig. 76

Routes of invasion of secondary acquired cholesteatoma of the attic

Secondary acquired cholesteatomas originate from a posterosuperior defect of the pars tensa or through a perforation in the Shrapnell membrane. They invade the attic, remaining lateral or medial to the malleus and incus. The medial route *(broken line)* leads through a triangular space situated between chorda tympani, malleus neck and long process of the incus. The lateral route *(solid line)* follows the lateral surface of the incus and malleus. In extensive lesions, lateral and medial routes of invasion are combined.

4. Surgical Treatment of Acquired Cholesteatoma

Aims

- Eradication of disease
- Prevention of recurrent and retention cholesteatomas
- Formation of a dry and self-cleansing cavity
- Restoration of tympanic aeration
- Reconstruction of a sound-transformer mechanism

Surgical Concepts

a) Closed (intact canal wall) Tympanomastoidectomy

The principle of the *intact canal wall tympanomastoidectomy* is to completely remove the cholesteatoma matrix without disturbing the anatomy of the external bony canal. The combined transcanal and transmastoid approach permits removal of cholesteatoma invading the facial recess. Cholesteatoma in the sinus tympani may be difficult to extirpate because of the limited visibility in this area.

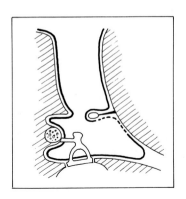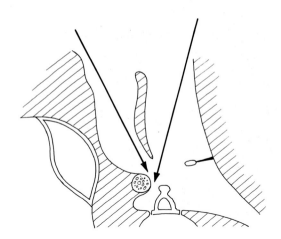

COMBINED TRANSCANAL + TRANSMASTOID APPROACH WITH POSTERIOR TYMPANOTOMY

Fig. 77

Principle of closed (intact canal wall) tympanomastoidectomy

The insert shows squamous epithelium *(solid line)* invading the middle ear cavity through a marginal perforation. Only a small remnant of mucosa *(broken line)* has remained under the anterior drum. The principle of a closed cavity (intact canal wall) mastoidectomy is to remove the matrix from the cavum tympani and mastoid working on both sides of the preserved bony canal wall.

b) Open (canal wall down) Tympanomastoidectomy

The priniciple of an open tympanomas-toidectomy is to create a large cavity in which no retention of keratinizing epithelium is possible. The drawback of a *classic radical mas-toidectomy* (open cavity without tympano-plasty) is the recurrent infection of the middle ear cavity through the perforated drum. Closure of the middle ear space by means of a tympanoplasty *(modified radical mastoidectomy)* eliminates the possible post-operative drainage from the middle ear, but there is insufficient attention to the elimina-tion of disease from the attic. The surgical technique *open cavity* presented on the follow-ing pages is characterized by the radical ex-enteration and exteriorization of both mas-toid and epitympanum (attic). The advan-tages of this technique, called *open mastoido-epitympanectomy with tympanoplasty (OMET)*, are the elimination of recurrent and residual disease as well as the formation of a dry and self-cleansing cavity.

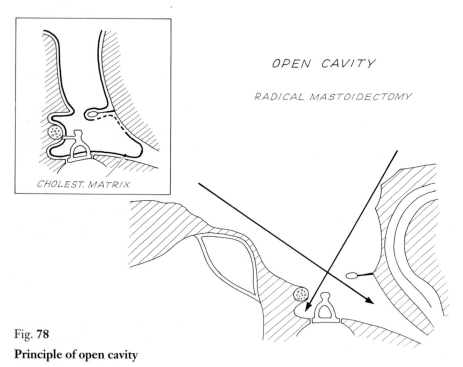

OPEN CAVITY

RADICAL MASTOIDECTOMY

CHOLEST. MATRIX

Fig. **78**

Principle of open cavity

The principle of a classic radical mastoidectomy is to include the external canal in a large open cavity. No tympanoplasty is performed.

c) Temporary Resection of the Canal Wall

Temporary resection of the canal wall gives the additional exposure of the tympanomas-toid space. The drawback is, however, the in-sufficient exteriorization and possible recur-rence of disease (including cholesteatoma) in the presence of persisting eustachian tube dysfunction. The technique of temporary re-section of the canal wall may also be called "open-closed" mastoidectomy.

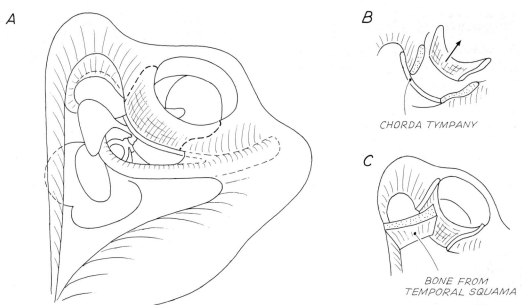

CHORDA TYMPANY

BONE FROM
TEMPORAL SQUAMA

Fig. 79

Temporary resection of the canal wall

A: The broken line shows the planes of resection of the posterosuperior canal wall. The oblique margin adds stability when replacing the bone.

B: Removal of the posterosuperior canal wall lateral to the chorda tympani.

C: The reconstructed canal wall may be stabilized with bone removed from the temporal squama (see Figs. 55 A–F), bone paste (bone dust and fibrin glue) as well as Ionomeric cement (Ionocap)*

d) Choice of Approach

The choice between open and closed tympanomastoidectomy depends on:

– *Function of the eustachian tube*
– *Extent of the disease*

The *pneumatization* of the temporal bone is a good measure of the function of the eustachian tube. A sclerotic mastoid is generally the result of poor eustachian tube function during childhood. The criteria for the choice of the approach in mastoid surgery are:

1. Limited disease with good pneumatization: *closed cavity*
2. Sclerotic mastoid with extensive disease: *open cavity*
3. Disease, particularly cholesteatoma matrix, cannot be radically removed beyond doubt: *open cavity*

The consistent application of these rules has significantly reduced the number of intact canal wall procedures performed in our department through the years (Table **15**).

Table **15** Frequency of closed and open cavities in surgery for cholesteatoma (1970–1976, n = 309)

	n	%
Closed cavity	225	73.0
Intact canal wall	210	68.0
Temporary resection of canal wall	15	5.0
Open cavity	84	27.0
Modified radical mastoidectomy	80	26.0
Radical mastoidectomy	4	1.3

* Ionos, Medizinische Produkte, GmbH, 82229 Seefeld, Germany

Specific Surgical Techniques for Cholesteatoma Removal

1. Closed Mastoido-Epitympanectomy with Tympanoplasty (closed MET)

Surgical Technique

The closed mastoido-epitympanectomy with tympanoplasty is a tympanomastoidectomy in which particular emphasis is applied to the work in the attic. A closed MET includes mastoidectomy, epitympanectomy, posterior tympanotomy, and tympanoplasty.

Surgical Highlights

- General anesthesia
- Retroauricular skin incision
- Meatal skin flap
- Canalplasty
- Middle ear inspection
- Mastoidectomy
- Epitympanectomy
- Posterior tympanotomy
- Complete removal of cholesteatoma matrix
- Tympanoplasty

Surgical Steps

The first surgical steps of intact canal MET are similar to those of retroauricular tympanoplasty.

- *Retroauricular skin incision* (Fig. **9 A**, p. 19)
- *Raising of periosteal flap* (Fig. **9 B**, p. 19)
- *Canal incisions* (Figs. **9 C**, p. 19, **D**, p. 20)
- *Exposure of external auditory canal and mastoid* (Figs. **9 E, F**, p. 20)
- *Elevation of meatal skin flap* (Fig. **9 G–L**, p. 21–22)
- *Canalplasty* (Figs. **9 M–P**, p. 23)

A

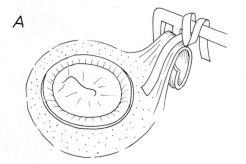

Fig. **80 A**

Surgical site after canalplasty

All bony overhang has been eliminated. The shape of the canal is that of an inverted truncated cone. A correct canalplasty facilitates tympanic membrane grafting, speeds up healing, ensures the self-cleansing property of the external canal, and makes it easier to carry out second-stage tympanoplasty.

Fig. 80 B

Middle ear inspection

The tympanomeatal flap is raised and the extent of cholesteatoma invasion of the middle ear assessed. The decision to perform a closed cavity is made on the basis of: (1) no evidence of eustachian tube dysfunction, (2) good pneumatization of the tympanomastoid cleft, and (3) limited extension of cholesteatoma.

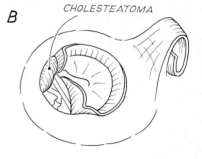

B   CHOLESTEATOMA

Fig. 80 C

Division of the incudostapedial joint

This step is necessary to avoid inducing a sensorineural hearing loss when working along the incus and malleus in the attic. In most instances, the long process of the incus is already eroded by the cholesteatoma so that division of the incudostapedial joint is superfluous.

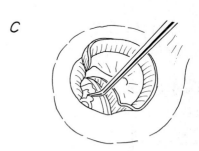

C

Mastoidectomy

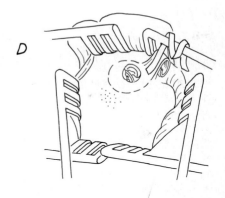

D

Fig. 80 D

Mastoidectomy: exposure of mastoid plane

The mastoid plane is exposed with two articulated retractors supplemented by a third rigid retractor placed between the temporalis muscle and mastoid tip.

Fig. 80 E

Mastoidectomy: identification of antrum

The antrum is identified at the intersection of two grooves formed by removing bone along the superior and posterior canal wall. The entrance of the bony external canal *should not* be lowered when drilled for the antrum (see Fig. 80 F). This is why the canalplasty should be completed *before* looking for the antrum. The middle fossa dura and sigmoid sinus are skeletonized at this stage when working in a sclerotic mastoid.

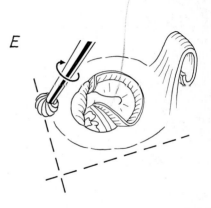

E

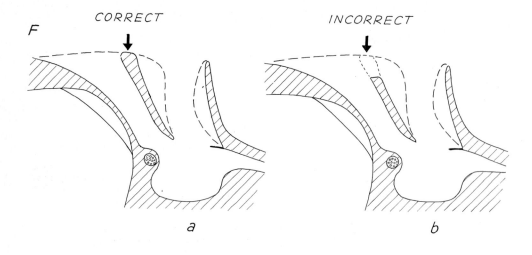

F

CORRECT

INCORRECT

a

b

Fig. **80 F**

Mastoidectomy: correct bone removal

a: The posterior canal wall should not be lowered during canalplasty and mastoidectomy.

b: Lowering the posterior entrance of the canal carries the risk of squamous epithelium ingrowth from the external canal into the mastoid (meatomastoid fistula).

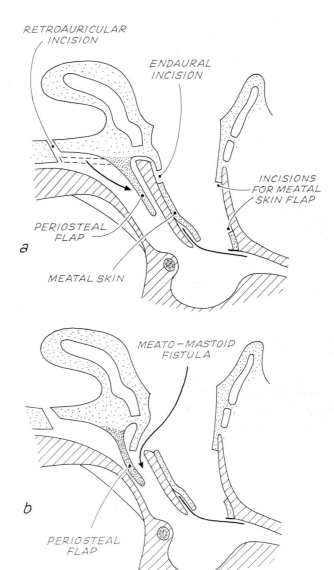

Fig. **80 G**

Mastoidectomy (cont.): danger of incorrect bone removal

Schematic cross section through the ear showing the correct (**a**) and incorrect (**b**) shaping of the posterior canal wall. Note that the posterior limb of the endaural incision must be made lower than the lateral entrance of the external canal and how the mastoid periosteal flap is rotated against the posterior canal wall to prevent atrophy of the bone and a meatomastoid fistula.

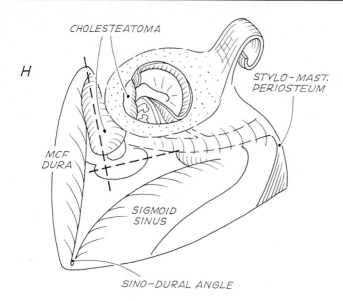

CHOLESTEATOMA

STYLO-MAST.
PERIOSTEUM

MCF
DURA

SIGMOID
SINUS

SINO-DURAL ANGLE

H

Fig. 80 H

Surgical site after mastoidectomy

The broken lines show the position of the antrum. The digastric ridge and the stylomastoid periosteum are exposed to identify the stylomastoid foramen. The course of the mastoid segment of the fallopian canal is identified through the bone using EMG monitoring of the facial muscles (NIM-2). The retrofacial cells are exenterated. The lateral and posterior semicircular canals are identified and the retrolabyrinthine cells exenterated. The sigmoid sinus and the middle cranial fossa dura are skeletonized.

EPITYMPANOTOMY (ATTICOTOMY)

I

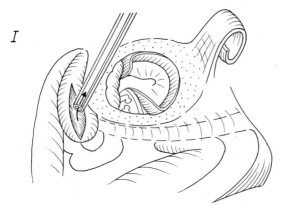

Fig. 80 I

Epitympanectomy: exposure of the attic

The lateral wall of the attic is removed with a diamond burr. The cholesteatoma fills the epitympanum. The matrix is opened with small tympanoplasty scissors, and the contents of the cholesteatoma sac are evacuated by suction. The size of the cholesteatoma is reduced to allow easier separation of the matrix from the surrounding bone.

Fig. **80 J**

Epitympanectomy: identification of tympanic facial nerve.

The atrophic incus is removed. The cholesteatoma matrix is elevated from the lateral semicircular canal. The tympanic facial nerve is identified along the inferior margin of the lateral semicircular canal. Only on rare occasions, does an extremely large cholesteatoma prevent adequate identification of the facial nerve along the lateral semicircular canal. In such a situation, it is best to follow the mastoid facial nerve from the stylomastoid foramen into the area where the anatomy has been distorted by the lesion. EMG monitoring of facial function (NIM-2) is essential in such a situation.

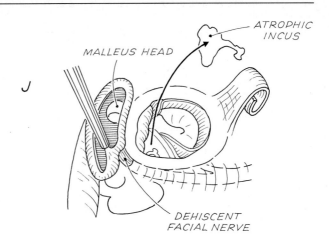

MALLEUS HEAD

ATROPHIC INCUS

DEHISCENT FACIAL NERVE

Fig. **80 K**

Management of semicircular canal fistula

a: Always expect a fistula when elevating the cholesteatoma matrix from the lateral semicircular canal. Look for a fistula before removing the medial wall of the cholesteatoma sac. In the presence of a fistula, leave the covering skin until the end of the operation to avoid damaging the inner ear.

b: Remove the skin over the fistula when the bone work and the removal of the remaining matrix is completed. Use constant irrigation. The matrix covering the fistula is only removed if the endostium is intact. This is usually possible in fistulas up to 2 mm in diameter. If the perilymphatic space is open, the skin covering the fistula is replaced in its original position.

c: If the matrix has been removed, the intact endostium of the fistula is covered with bone dust (obtained by drilling) mixed with fibrin glue (bone paste).

d: The fistula is finally covered with fresh temporalis fascia placed over the bone paste.

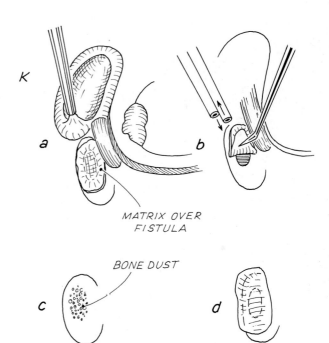

MATRIX OVER FISTULA

BONE DUST

CHORDA – TENSOR FOLD

CHOLESTEATOMA MATRIX

L

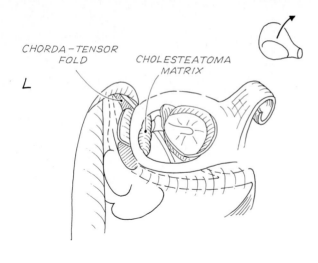

Fig. 80 L

Epitympanectomy (cont.): exenteration of the attic

The malleus neck is divided and the head of the malleus removed. The cholesteatoma matrix is carefully detached from the walls of the epitympanum, and the size of the cholesteatoma sac is successively reduced by cutting away excess matrix. The completely closed chorda–tensor fold is removed. The matrix lying lateral to the tympanic segment of the facial nerve is removed from the supralabyrinthine and supratubal recess. The position of the geniculum, petrosal nerve, and labyrinthine segment of the facial nerve should be known to avoid injury of a dehiscent nerve. A spontaneous dehiscence of the facial nerve may exist proximal to the geniculum. EMG monitoring of the facial muscles with the NIM-2 is very helpful in this phase of surgery to avoid causing a lesion of the facial nerve.

POSTERIOR TYMPANOTOMY

M

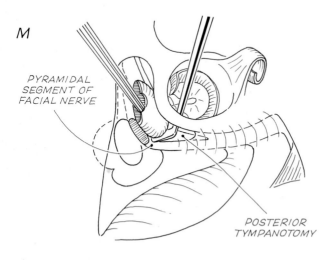

PYRAMIDAL SEGMENT OF FACIAL NERVE

POSTERIOR TYMPANOTOMY

Fig. 80 M

Posterior tympanotomy

The bone situated between the pyramidal facial nerve and the chorda tympani is drilled away along the tympanic segment of the fallopian canal. The resulting opening to the middle ear is the posterior tympanotomy. A lesion of the facial nerve should not occur because the posterior tympanotomy is carried out under direct visual control of the nerve and with EMG monitoring of the facial muscles (NIM-2). The size of the tympanotomy depends on the extent of the cholesteatoma in the facial recess and sinus tympani. A wide exposure of the sinus tympani requires sacrifice of the chorda. If the cholesteatoma is limited to the superior half of the oval window niche (above the stapes arch), complete removal of the matrix can be accomplished at this stage, working from both sides of the intact canal wall (combined approach).

Fig. **80 N**

Posterior tympanotomy: removal of cholesteatoma from the oval window

Matrix covering the stapes and oval window is removed after completion of all bone work because uncontrolled suction irrigation might damage the exposed inner ear.

a: The last portion of cholesteatoma invading the oval window niche between the stapes arch and facial nerve is exposed.

b: The removal of the matrix from the oval window begins anteriorly where the footplate (or membrane covering the oval window) is best identified. For the elevation of matrix from the oval window, the same precautions should be taken as when working over a fistula of the lateral semicircular canal (see Fig. 80 K, p.159).

c: The posterior matrix is best removed through the transcanal approach. Drilling a small notch in the posterior canal wall may be necessary to visualize the posterior footplate. Removal of matrix from the stapes is performed in a posteroanterior direction, taking advantage of the stability offered by the stapedial tendon.

d: The matrix has been completely removed from the oval window niche and stapes. The notch in the posterior canal wall will be reconstructed later on with preserved septal or tragal cartilage. Cutting the stapes arch with crurotomy scissors to remove matrix surrounding the stapes arch is rarely necessary. Manipulations around the stapes arch require caution to avoid luxation of the footplate.

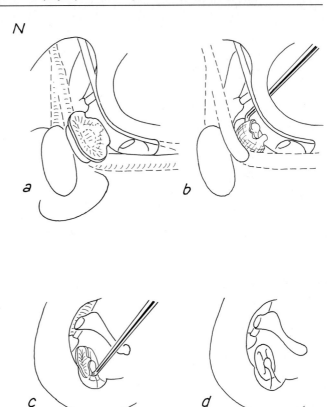

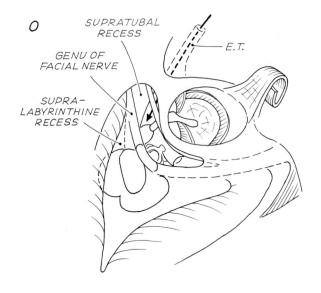

O

SUPRATUBAL
RECESS

E.T.

GENU OF
FACIAL NERVE

SUPRA-
LABYRINTHINE
RECESS

Fig. 80 O

Surgical site following completion of closed tympanomastoidectomy

The supralabyrinthine and supratubal recesses are exenterated. Good knowledge of the anatomy of the tympanic and labyrinthine segment of the facial nerve is necessary for this purpose. Keep in mind the acute angle formed by the tympanic and labyrinthine facial nerve and that the proximal labyrinthine segment of the fallopian canal is nearly covered by the lateral tympanic segment. Note that the chorda–tensor fold was removed to provide adequate ventilation of the anterior attic (*arrow*).

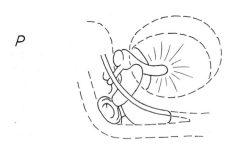

P

Fig. 80 P

Tympanoplasty

Primary reconstruction of the ossicular chain is possible in this case because the stapes, the malleus handle, the tensor tympani tendon, and the pars tensa of the tympanic membrane are intact. A modified Ionomer incus is interposed between the stapes head and malleus handle (see also Figs. 22 J–M). If the malleus handle is missing, the reconstruction of the ossicular chain is carried out at a second stage.

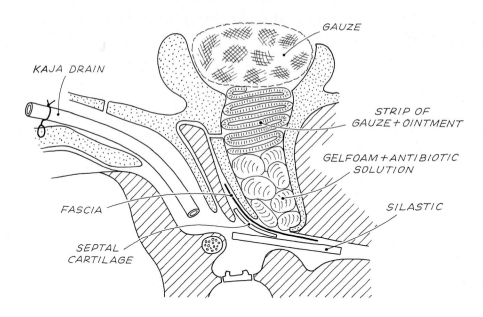

Fig. **81**

Packing and transmastoid drain

Schematic representation of packing and transmastoid drain in closed mastoido-epitympanectomy with tympanoplasty. For the sake of demonstration, a different ossicular situation from that of Fig. 80 P is illustrated. The malleus handle and the stapes arch are missing. A first-stage tympanoplasty was performed. Silastic sheeting was introduced into the tympanic cavity and eustachian tube because of the defective middle ear mucosa. Septal cartilage is used to reconstruct the posterior canal wall. An anterior underlay of temporalis fascia was used to reconstruct the tympanic membrane. Gelfoam pledgets impregnated with Otosporin keep the meatal skin and the underlaid fascia in position over the tympanic sulcus. The external canal is packed with a strip of gauze impregnated with antibiotic ointment (Terracortril). The concha is covered by a large gauze. A conventional pressure dressing is applied over the wound.

2. Open Mastoido-Epitympanectomy with Tympanoplasty (open MET)

Surgical Technique

The surgical principles of an open cavity are

1. *Radical exenteration* of tympanomastoid cell tracts, and

2. *Adequate exteriorization* of the surgical cavity.

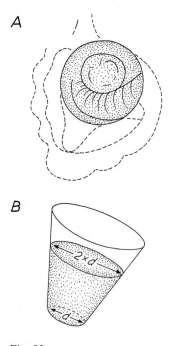

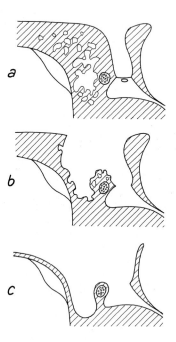

Fig. **82**

Adequate exteriorization of open cavity

Adequate exteriorization implies shaping the open cavity as an inverted truncated cone with a lateral diameter twice the size of the medial diameter. The cavity volume is reduced by removing the largest amount of lateral bone.

A: Axial view of open cavity. Note that the bottom of the cavity includes the grafted part of the meso- and hypotympanum as well as the exteriorized epitympanum. The lateral entrance of the cavity extends from the tympanic bone (anteroinferiorly) to the skeletonized middle cranial fossa dura (superiorly) and the facial ridge (posteriorly).

B: Open cavity showing the reduction in volume obtained by the lateral removal of bone.

Fig. **83**

Mastoidectomy: correct exenteration and exteriorization

a: Schematic view of mastoid air cells.

b: Insufficient exenteration and exteriorization of mastoid air cells.

c: Correct exenteration and exteriorization of mastoid. All pneumatic cells are removed. The lateral bone is lowered over and behind the sigmoid sinus and the mastoid facial nerve. There is no bony overhang of the anterior canal wall.

Fig. **84**

Epitympanectomy: correct exenteration and exteriorization (cont.)

a: Schematic showing the supralabyrinthine air cells.

b: Schematic view following correct exenteration and exteriorization of the epitympanum. The middle cranial fossa dura as well as the tympanic and labyrinthine segments of the facial nerve are skeletonized. The malleus head has been removed to exteriorize the attic.

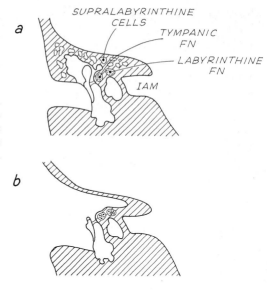

Fig. **85**

Surgical anatomy of the epitympanum

The medial wall of the attic is divided by the geniculum of the facial nerve in the *supralabyrinthine recess* (posteriorly) and the *supratubal recess* (sinus epitympani) anteriorly. The supratubal recess is limited by the semicanal of the tensor tympani muscle, by the geniculum and tympanic segments of the facial nerve, and by the root of the zygoma. Although the supratubal recess is well known, no mention of the supralabyrinthine recess is found in the literature. The *supralabyrinthine recess* is limited by the tympanic and labyrinthine segments of the facial nerve, the middle cranial fossa dura, and the bony superior and lateral ampullae. This space is frequently involved in chronic infections and may be the source of continuous secretion if not adequately exenterated and exteriorized.

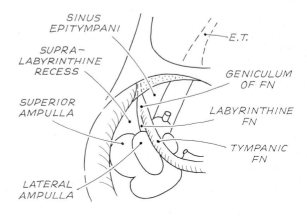

Surgical Highlights

- Retroauricular skin incision
- Meatal skin flap
- Canalplasty
- Wide removal of bone over middle cranial fossa dura, sigmoid sinus, and sinus dura angle
- Exposure of digastric muscle
- Identification of stylomastoid foramen along stylomastoid periosteum
- Epitympanotomy with identification of tympanic segment of the facial nerve
- Lowering of facial ridge over mastoid segment of the fallopian canal

- Radical exenteration and exposure of retrofacial and retrolabyrinthine cells
- Radical exenteration and exposure of supralabyrinthine and supratubal recesses
- Extended canalplasty with removal of anteroinferior overhang of tympanic bone
- Radical removal of remnant matrix from tympanic cavity
- Formation of a new tympanic sulcus
- Removal of mastoid tip
- Tympanoplasty
- Obliteration of posterior cavity with myosubcutaneous occipital flap

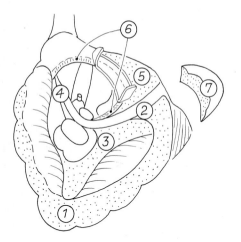

Fig. **86**

Checklist for bone work in open MET

The recommended sequence of bone removal for an open MET is:

1. Wide lateral bone removal over root of the zygoma with skeletonization of middle cranial fossa dura, sigmoid sinus, digastric ridge, and stylomastoid foramen

2. Identification of the tympanic segment of the fallopian canal and lowering of facial ridge

3. Radical exenteration and exteriorization of the retrofacial and retrolabyrinthine cells.

4. Radical exenteration and exteriorization of the epitympanum (supralabyrinthine and supratubal recesses)

5. Extended anteroinferior canalplasty

6. Formation of a new tympanic sulcus

7. Removal of mastoid tip

Surgical Steps

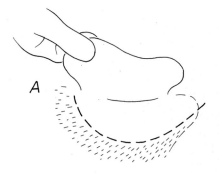

Fig. 87 A

Retroauricular skin incision

The retroauricular skin incision is carried out along the hairline and extends inferiorly over the mastoid tip into a crease of the skin. The skin incision must be posterior enough to avoid lying over the exenterated mastoid bone.

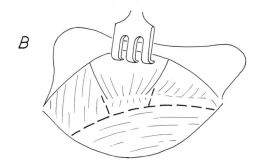

Fig. 87 B

Exposure of the mastoid

The soft tissues are elevated over the mastoid. The periosteum covering the mastoid is incised from the posterior edge of the temporalis muscle to the mastoid tip. Two small anterior incisions are performed along the superior and inferior edge of the external canal.

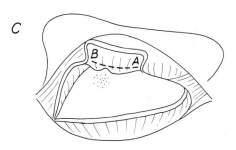

Fig. 87 C

Exposure of the external auditory canal

The posterior wall of the external auditory canal is incised (*A–B*) with a No. 15 blade, remaining a few millimeters deeper than Henle's spine (see also Fig. 80 G).

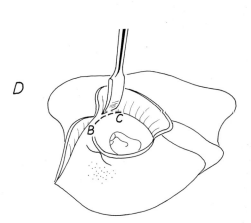

Fig. 87 D

Exposure of external auditory canal (cont.)

The external canal incision is extended anteriorly to 2 o'clock (*broken line, B–C*). A Key raspatory is used to elevate the canal skin exposing the root of the zygoma.

E

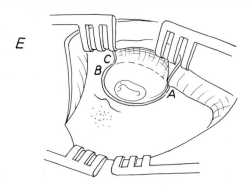

Fig. 87 E

Exposure of external auditory canal (cont.)

Two articulated retroauricular retractors are introduced, exposing the external canal. The posterior (*A–B*) and the anterior (*B–C*) limbs of the canal incisions are shown.

F

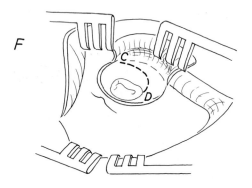

Fig. 87 F

Meatal skin flap

An ascending spiral incision (*D–C*) is made with a No. 11 blade, meeting the anterior limb of the canal incision (*C*).

G

Fig. 87 G

Meatal skin flap (cont.)

A "universal" microraspatory is used to elevate the skin from the bony canal wall.

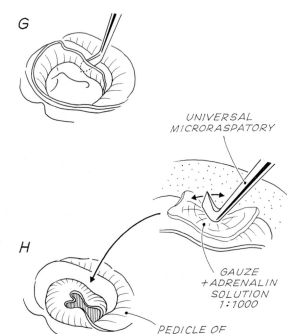

UNIVERSAL
MICRORASPATORY

GAUZE
+ADRENALIN
SOLUTION
1:1000

PEDICLE OF
MEATAL SKIN

Fig. 87 H

Meatal skin flap (cont.)

The lateral canal skin is elevated under direct vision to the tympanic sulcus (posteriorly) and to the edge of the anteroinferior bony overhang. A small piece of gauze soaked in Adrenalin (1:1000) facilitates elevation of the meatal skin. Bleeding during elevation of the meatal skin flap is greatly reduced by infiltrating the canal skin with local anesthesia at the time of the retroauricular skin incision.

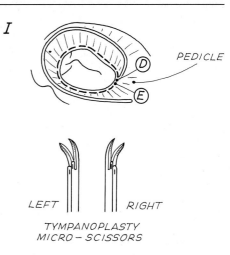

Fig. 87 I

Meatal skin flap (cont.)

A medial circular incision of the meatal skin
(*D–E*) is carried out, remaining 2 mm lateral to
the visible fibrous tympanic annulus and at the
level of the bony overhang of the anteroinferior
canal wall. Straight, as well as curved *(right and
left)*, tympanoplasty microscissors are used to in-
cise the mobilized meatal skin.

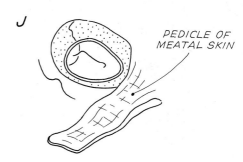

Fig. 87 J

Meatal skin flap (cont.)

The mobilized meatal skin is elevated out of the
bony canal, forming an inferiorly pedicled flap.

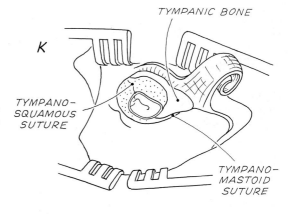

Fig. 87 K

Meatal skin flap (cont.)

The complete tympanic ring is exposed by elevating the lateral canal skin between tympanomastoid and tympanosquamous sutures.

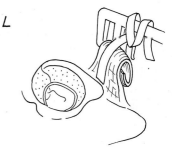

Fig. 87 L

Meatal skin flap (cont.)

The meatal skin flap is secured by means of a
malleable aluminum strip to the retroauricular
retractor.

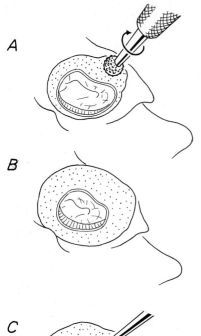

A

Fig. 88 A

Canalplasty

The bony external canal is widened, using sharp and diamond burrs until the edge of the medial meatal skin is reached.

B

Fig. 88 B

Canalplasty (cont.)

View of the external canal following lateral widening.

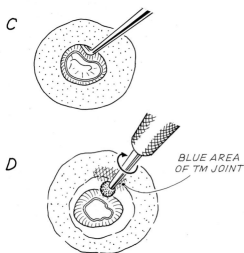

C

Fig. 88 C

Canalplasty (cont.)

The medial sleeve of canal skin is elevated from the bone using a universal microdissector (see also Fig. 87 H). The skin elevation is done step-by-step in conjunction with the continuous removal of overhanging bone.

D

BLUE AREA OF TM JOINT

Fig. 88 D

Canalplasty (cont.)

Care is taken not to break into the temporomandibular joint when widening the anterior canal wall. The bone removal is stopped when a pink-blue discoloration appears through the bone over the temporomandibular joint. Note that irrigation enhances the transparency of bone.

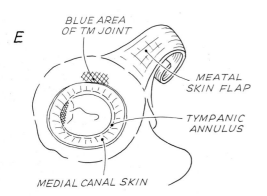

E

BLUE AREA OF TM JOINT

MEATAL SKIN FLAP

TYMPANIC ANNULUS

MEDIAL CANAL SKIN

Fig. 88 E

Canalplasty (cont.)

Widening of the bony external canal is stopped when the complete fibrous tympanic annulus is visualized with one position of the microscope. At this stage, the canal has the form of an inverted truncated cone (see. Fig. 82). All bony overhang is eliminated to assure the self-cleansing capacity of the external ear.

Fig. **89**

Exploration of the middle ear

Following completion of the canal-plasty, a posterosuperior tympano-meatal flap is elevated to assess the intratympanic extent of cholesteatoma invasion and the condition of the ossicular chain. In the presented case, the cholesteatoma covers the oval window niche above the chorda tympani and has eroded the long process of the incus.

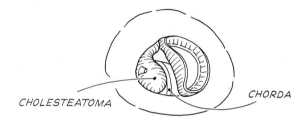

CHOLESTEATOMA   CHORDA

Fig. **90 A**

Antrotomy (atticotomy)

Two grooves are drilled along the superior and posterior canal walls. The antrum is located at the intersection of both grooves.

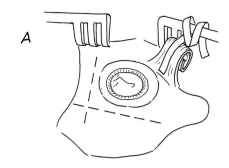

A

Fig. **90 B**

Antrotomy (cont.)

The cholesteatoma fills the antrum. The lateral wall of the attic is drilled away *(epitympanotomy)*. The decision to perform an open cavity is made on the basis of
1. history of poor eustachian tube function,
2. reduced pneumatization of the mastoid, and
3. extent of cholesteatoma invasion.

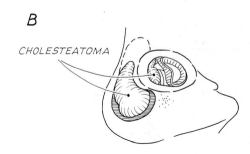

B

CHOLESTEATOMA

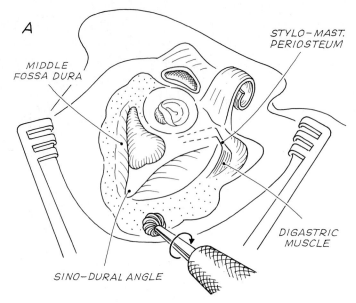

A

MIDDLE
FOSSA DURA

STYLO—MAST.
PERIOSTEUM

DIGASTRIC
MUSCLE

SINO—DURAL ANGLE

Fig. **91 A**

Mastoidectomy: wide removal of lateral bone

A third retroauricular retractor is used to expose the temporal squama and the mastoid tip. A wide removal of bone (step 1 of checklist, see Fig. 86) is carried out from the zygomatic arch to the middle fossa dura, the sino-dural angle, the sigmoid sinus, and the digastric muscle. The stylomastoid periosteum is followed to the stylomastoid foramen. EMG monitoring of facial function (NIM-2) is helpful when drilling close to the stylomastoid foramen.

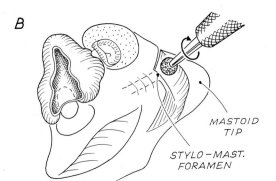

B

MASTOID
TIP

STYLO—MAST.
FORAMEN

Fig. **91 B**

Mastoidectomy: exposure of the stylo-mastoid foramen

This is step 2 of the check list in Fig. 86. Progressive removal of bone along the stylomastoid periosteum leads to the identification of the stylomastoid foramen. At this stage, a crack forms lateral to the stylomastoid foramen, mobilizing the complete mastoid tip. EMG monitoring of facial function (NIM-2) is very helpful during this step of the procedure.

Fig. 91 C

Mastoidectomy: exposure of the tympanic facial nerve

The tympanic fallopian canal is identified at the inferior edge of the lateral semicircular canal. Remember to expect a possible perilymph fistula when elevating the matrix from the lateral semicircular canal, even if the patient had no preoperative vertigo (see also Fig. 80 K).

a: Position of the tympanic facial nerve at the inferior edge of the lateral canal.

b: The universal microraspatory is the ideal instrument for elevating the cholesteatoma matrix from a dehiscent facial nerve. EMG monitoring of facial function (NIM-2) is very helpful during this stage of the procedure.

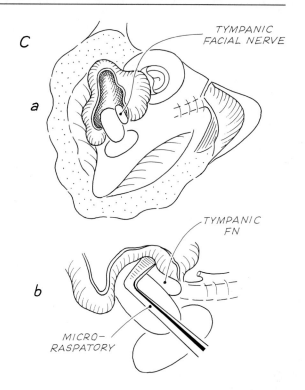

Fig. 91 D

Mastoidectomy: lowering the facial ridge

Lowering the facial ridge is performed with diamond burrs and suction-irrigation from both ends, the tympanic segment of the facial nerve, and the stylomastoid foramen. The bone is removed until the nerve becomes visible under the last eggshell of bone.

a: The level of the mastoid segment of the fallopian canal is determined by a line drawn from the tympanic facial nerve to the stylomastoid foramen.

b: A further landmark for the mastoid facial nerve is the inferior edge of the posterior semicircular canal. The pyramidal segment of the facial nerve is situated 2 mm anteriorly and laterally to the inferior edge of the posterior semicircular canal.

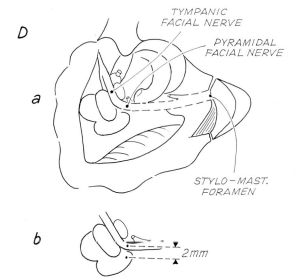

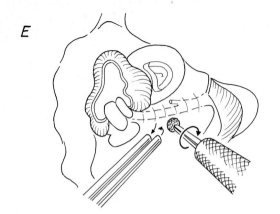

E

Fig. 91 E

Mastoidectomy: exenteration and exteriorization of the retrofacial cells

This is step 3 of the checklist in Fig. 86. The retrofacial cells are completely removed, keeping the skeletonized facial nerve in view. The rotation of the burr is away from the facial nerve. Complete exenteration of the retrofacial cells may require exposure of the blue area of the jugular bulb medial to the mastoid segment of the fallopian canal.

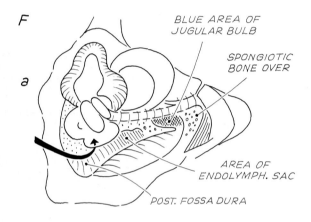

F

a

BLUE AREA OF
JUGULAR BULB

SPONGIOTIC
BONE OVER

AREA OF
ENDOLYMPH. SAC

POST. FOSSA DURA

Fig. 91 F

Mastoidectomy: exenteration and exteriorization of the retrolabyrinthine cells

This is step 4 of the checklist in Fig. 86. The radical exenteration of the retrolabyrinthine cells requires skeletonization of the semicircular canals.

a: Correct exteriorization of cells extending medial to the posterior canal is impossible.

b: Exenterated cells below the posterior semicircular canal must be obliterated with the suboccipital myosubcutaneous flap for correct exteriorization of the open cavity.

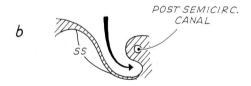

POST SEMICIRC.
CANAL

b

SS

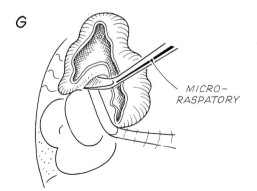

G

MICRO-
RASPATORY

Fig. 91 G

Epitympanectomy

This is step 4 of the checklist in Fig. 86. The cholesteatoma matrix is elevated from the supralabyrinthine and supratubal recesses, remaining lateral to the tympanic segment of the facial nerve. The matrix invading the oval window niche is left temporarily in situ.

Fig. 91 H

Epitympanectomy (cont.): radical exentera-tion and exteriorization of the supralabyrin-thine and supratubal recesses

Following removal of the matrix, the supralabyrin-thine and supratubal recesses are exenterated, using diamond burrs with suction-irrigation. The rotation of the burr is reversed when working along the tympanic and labyrinthine segments of the facial nerve. Correct exteriorization of the attic requires wide removal of the root of the zygo-matic arch and skeletonization of the middle fossa dura.

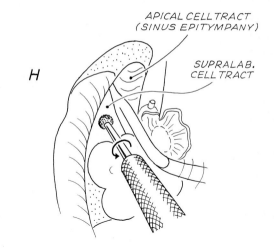

Fig. 91 I

Epitympanectomy (cont.): radical ex-enteration and exteriorization of the supralabyrinthine and supratubal recesses

a: Surgical site following correct epitym-panectomy.

b: The radical exenteration of the medial wall of the attic requires precise anatomical knowledge of this area. The supralabyrin-thine recess is limited inferiorly by the laby-rinthine and tympanic segments of the fal-lopian canal, superiorly by the middle cranial fossa dura, and posteriorly by the bony superior and lateral ampullae (see also Figs. 84 and 85).

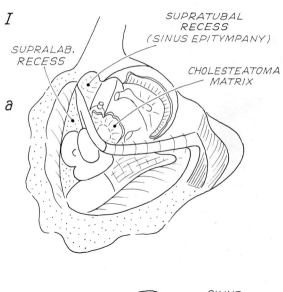

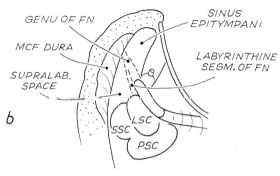

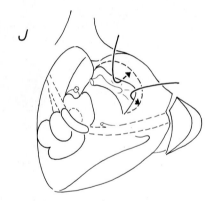

Fig. **91 J**

Extended canalplasty

This is step 5 of the checklist in Fig. 86. The anteroinferior overhang of the external canal must be eliminated for correct exteriorization.

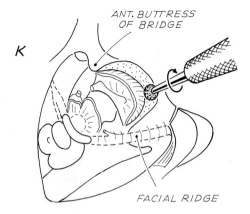

ANT. BUTTRESS
OF BRIDGE

FACIAL RIDGE

Fig. **91 K**

Extended canalplasty (cont.)

The medial sleeve of anterior–inferior meatal skin is elevated away from the bone. The excess bone is removed with diamond burrs until the fibrous tympanic annulus becomes visible with one position of the microscope. Care is taken not to break through the bone into the temporomandibular joint (see also Fig. 88 D). The anterior buttress of the canal bridge is removed to the level of the attic.

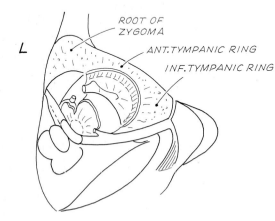

ROOT OF
ZYGOMA

ANT. TYMPANIC RING

INF. TYMPANIC RING

Fig. **91 L**

Extended canalplasty (cont.)

Correct exteriorization of the open cavity after extensive removal of bone over the root of the zygoma and of the anterior tympanic ring. The inferior tympanic ring is lowered to the level of the stylomastoid foramen.

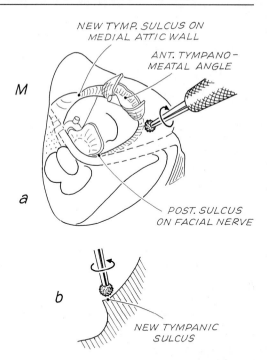

Fig. **91 M**

New tympanic sulcus

This is step 6 of the checklist in Fig. 86.

a: The anterior remnant of tympanic membrane with adjacent meatal skin is elevated to identify the original tympanic sulcus (at 2 o'clock and 5 o'clock). A new tympanic sulcus is drilled for support of the fascial graft superiorly (anterior attic) and inferoposteriorly to the level of the stapedial muscle and tendon, just in front of the pyramidal segment of the fallopian canal.

b: The new tympanic "sulcus" is indeed a "ledge" drilled into the bony canal wall.

Fig. **91 N**

New tympanic sulcus (cont.)

If there is no tympanic membrane remnant, the new bony sulcus is carried out circumferentially from the semicanal of the tensor tympani muscle (1 o'clock) to the pyramidal process (10 o'clock). The new "ledge" of bone will support the fascial overlay.

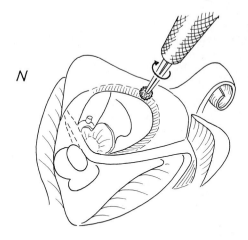

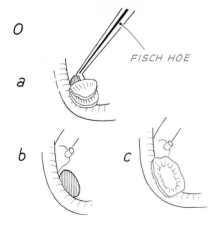

FISCH HOE

Fig. 91 O

Removal of cholesteatoma from oval window

The cholesteatoma matrix covering the oval window niche is removed after completion of the bone work to avoid the risk of prolonged exposure of the inner ear. Repair of a perilymphatic fistula is dangerous if it is followed by major bone work involving continuous suction-irrigation.

a: The elevation of matrix covering the oval window is started at the anterior edge using a 0.2-mm footplate elevator.

b: The matrix is removed, leaving intact the tiny membrane covering the oval window. The matrix is left in place if its removal would imply wide exposure of the perilymphatic space. In this situation, a type IV tympanoplasty or a second-stage tympanoplasty with delayed removal of matrix would be performed to avoid the danger of labyrinthitis.

c: The oval window is covered with pressed tragal perichondrium after complete removal of the matrix.

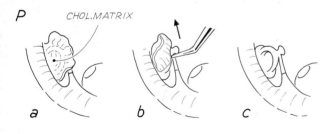

CHOL.MATRIX

Fig. 91 P

Removal of cholesteatoma from oval window (cont.)

a: The cholesteatoma covers the intact stapes arch.

b: The matrix is degloved from the stapes arch, working in posteroanterior direction and taking advantage of the stability afforded by the stapedial tendon.

c: The matrix is removed without lesion of the annular ligament. Luxation of the stapes footplate carries a high risk of inner ear trauma or labyrinthitis. In rare cases, radical extirpation of the matrix requires removal of the stapes arch with crurotomy scissors.

Fig. 91 Q

Removal of cholesteatoma from the round window

a: The matrix covers the round window niche.

b: The elevation of the matrix is started from the promontory and carried out under direct vision to the entrance of the niche.

c: Separation of the matrix from the round window membrane should be made under direct vision. This requires removal of the upper edge of the round window niche with a diamond drill until the round window membrane is exposed.

d: The matrix has been completely stripped from the round window membrane without rupture.

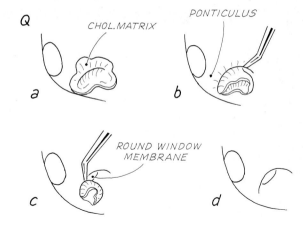

Fig. 91 R

Removal of mastoid tip

This is step 7 of the checklist in Fig. 86. The mastoid tip is removed before grafting because it may involve hemorrhage from small arteries surrounding the stylomastoid foramen.

a: The fracture line lateral to the stylomastoid foramen (see Fig. 91 B) is enlarged with a diamond drill for better mobilization of the mastoid tip.

b: The mobilized mastoid tip is grasped with a rongeur and rotated outward in a clockwise manner.

c: The medial surface of the mastoid tip is peeled away from the digastric muscle, continuing the clockwise rotation of the rongeur. Strong scissors are used to cut the remaining attachments to the stylomastoid muscle, working away from the stylomastoid foramen. Bleeding vessels are coagulated bipolarly.

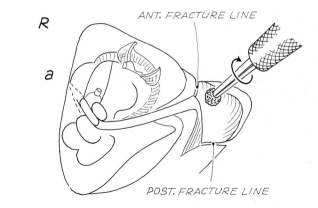

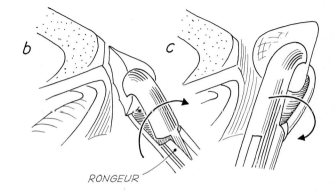

3. Tympanoplasty in Open Mastoido-Epitympanectomy

Tympanoplasty in an open cavity varies depending on the amount of residual tympanic membrane. *Underlay grafting* is used in the presence of an anterior remnant of the drum. *Overlay grafting* is the technique of choice when no anterior tympanic membrane remnant is present. Both techniques are discussed separately.

3.1 Anterior Underlay Grafting

a) First-Stage Tympanoplasty

This technique is used whenever immediate ossiculoplasty is not indicated. This is the case when the stapes arch is missing and the footplate is mobile or fixed. Here, the anterior underlay grafting is described for basic situation II (mobile footplate with malleus handle).

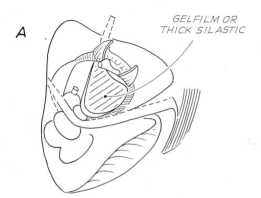

GELFILM OR
THICK SILASTIC

A

Fig. 92 A

Tympanotubal sheeting

Sheeting (see Fig. 49 A, B) is introduced into the cavum tympani and tympanic ostium of the eustachian tube because the mucosa of the middle ear is defective. Gelfilm is used instead of Silastic in the presence of an active middle ear infection.

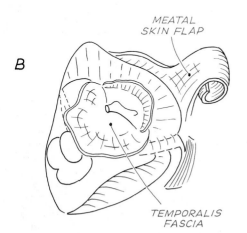

MEATAL
SKIN FLAP

B

TEMPORALIS
FASCIA

Fig. 92 B

Anterior underlay grafting

A piece of fresh temporalis fascia (see Fig. 14 G) is positioned under the anterior remnant of the tympanic membrane. Care is taken to place the posterior fascia over the new tympanic sulcus, as well as over the tympanic segment of the facial nerve and the semicanal of the tensor tympani muscle. The fascia should only extend a few millimeters onto the supporting ledge of bone because redundant fascia delays healing.

b) Type III Tympanoplasty

This type of tympanoplasty is carried out in the presence of an intact and mobile stapes (see basic situation III$_1$).

Fig. 93 A

Anterior fascial underlay

The fresh temporalis fascia is placed under the anterior remnant of the tympanic membrane. Contact with the lateral wall of the protympanum is maintained with sheeting (Gelfilm or Silastic) or with Gelfoam pledgets soaked in Ringer's solution. Inferiorly, the fascia lies over the new tympanic sulcus.

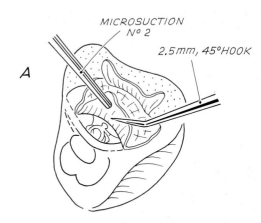

A

Fig. 93 B

Anterior fascial underlay (cont.)

Surgical site after anterior fascial underlay. Note that the stapes head is higher than the surrounding fascia (see also Fig. 40 B). The fascia covers the tympanic facial nerve in the semicanal of the tensor tympani muscle, extending only a few millimeters onto the new tympanic sulcus.

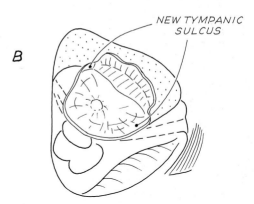

B

3.2 Overlay Grafting

This technique is used when there is no anterior remnant of the tympanic membrane.

a) Type IV Tympanoplasty

In the illustrated case, only the mobile footplate is present (basic situation III$_5$). An alternative to type IV tympanoplasty is a staged tympanoplasty (see Fig. 95).

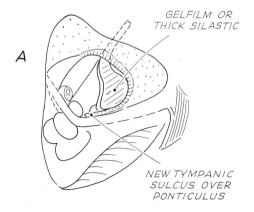

GELFILM OR
THICK SILASTIC

NEW TYMPANIC
SULCUS OVER
PONTICULUS

Fig. 94 A

Sheeting of the middle ear and the eustachian tube

The new bony tympanic sulcus goes from the anterior attic to the posterior edge of the oval window for adaptation of the graft at the lower border of the oval window. A thick Silastic sheet (or, in case of active infection, a Gelfilm) is placed in the hypotympanum and proximal eustachian tube.

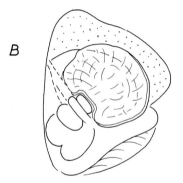

Fig. 94 B

Overlay of temporalis fascia

The fresh temporalis fascia is placed over the new tympanic sulcus and semicanal of the tensor tympani muscle. The fascia covers the round window niche and approaches the lower edge of the oval window.

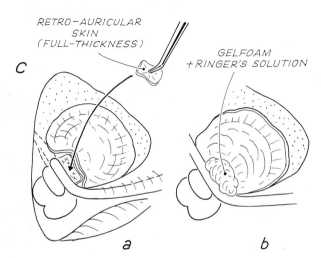

RETRO-AURICULAR
SKIN
(FULL-THICKNESS)

GELFOAM
+ RINGER'S SOLUTION

a   *b*

Fig. 94 C

Skin grafting of oval window

a: A small piece of full-thickness retroauricular skin is obtained with a No. 20 blade from the posterior surface of the auricle and transported over the mobile footplate.

b: A Gelfoam pledget soaked in Ringer's solution keeps the skin graft in position over the mobile footplate.

b) First-Stage Tympanoplasty

This type of tympanoplasty is used in the presence of the footplate (mobile or fixed) without other ossicles (basic situation III_5, III_6).

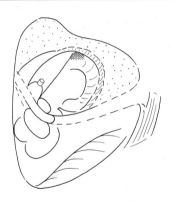

Fig. 95 A

New tympanic sulcus

The new tympanic sulcus is drilled from the anterior attic to the pyramidal process.

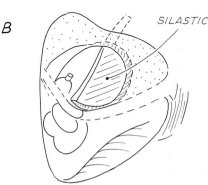

Fig. 95 B

Tubotympanic sheeting

Thick Silastic sheeting or (in case of active infection) a piece of Gelfilm is placed in the mesotympanum and hypotympanum, extending into the proximal eustachian tube. The sheeting covers the oval window.

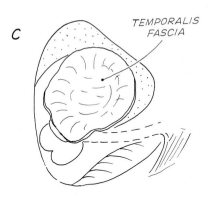

Fig. 95 C

Overlay of temporalis fascia

The fresh temporalis fascia is slightly larger than the tympanic sulcus and covers the semicanal of the tensor tympani, the lateral semicircular canal, and the new tympanic sulcus.

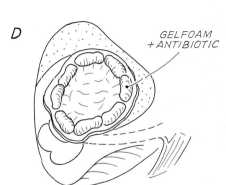

Fig. 95 D

Fixation of temporalis fascia

Gelfoam pledgets soaked in Otosporin keep the fascia in place.

4. Exteriorization of Open Cavity

POORLY PNEUMATIZED MASTOID

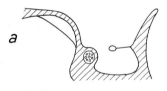

a

HIGHLY PNEUMATIZED MASTOID

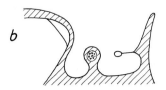

b

Fig. 96

Correct exteriorization of open cavity

Correct exteriorization of an open cavity requires a different technique depending upon the degree of pneumatization of the mastoid.

a: A poorly pneumatized mastoid is exteriorized by extensive bone removal over the facial nerve and sigmoid sinus.

b: In a highly pneumatized mastoid, the radical removal of the retrofacial and retrolabyrinthine cells may result in an insufficiently exteriorized cavity because of a prominent facial nerve and/or sigmoid sinus. In such a case, obliteration of the posterior cavity with a suboccipital myosubcutaneous flap is mandatory.

The exteriorization of the open cavity for poorly and highly pneumatized mastoids is described separately.

4.1 Poorly Pneumatized Mastoid

This case relates to basic situation II_1.

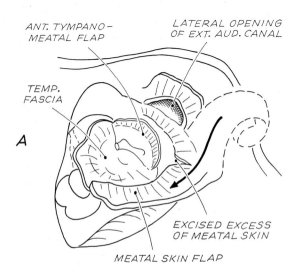

ANT. TYMPANO-MEATAL FLAP

LATERAL OPENING OF EXT. AUD. CANAL

TEMP. FASCIA

A

EXCISED EXCESS OF MEATAL SKIN

MEATAL SKIN FLAP

Fig. 97 A

Repositioning of meatal skin flap

The poorly pneumatized mastoid was adequately exteriorized by bone removal. The meatal skin flap is replaced, covering the posterior edge of the temporalis fascia. A triangle of meatal skin is excised with tympanoplasty scissors for better adaptation of the skin flap.

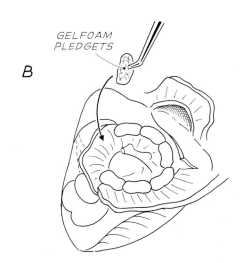

B

Fig. **97 B**

Fixation of overlaid fascia and meatal skin

Gelfoam pledgets soaked in Oto-sporin keep the temporalis fascia and meatal skin in place.

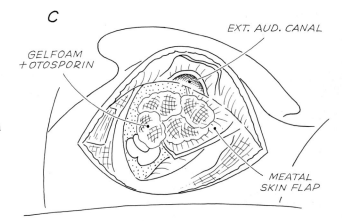

C

Fig. **97 C**

Packing of open cavity

The exteriorized cavity is filled with Gelfoam soaked in Otosporin.

4.2 Highly Pneumatized Mastoid

The exenteration of deep retrofacial and retrolabyrinthine cells prevents correct exteriorization of the posterior cavity. In this case, a myosubcutaneous occipital flap is used to obliterate the posterior cavity.

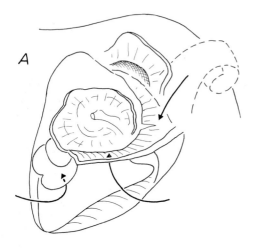

Fig. **98 A**

Replacement of meatal skin flap

The meatal skin is positioned over the posterior edge of the temporalis fascia. A triangle of skin is excised for better adaptation of the skin flap to the inferior cavity. The posterior arrows show the insufficiently exteriorized retrofacial and retrolabyrinthine cells.

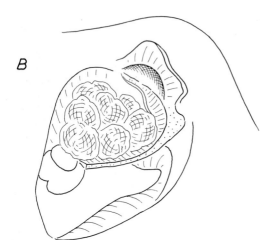

Fig. **98 B**

Anterior packing of open cavity

Gelfoam soaked in Otosporin fills the cavity, anterior to the meatal skin flap.

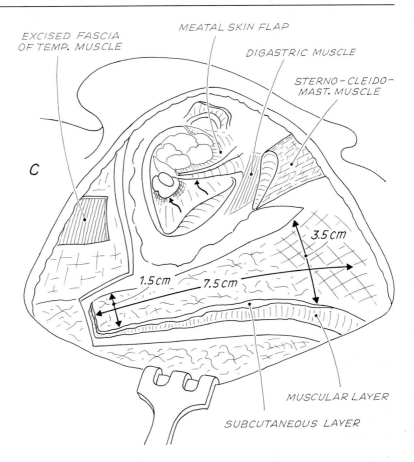

EXCISED FASCIA
OF TEMP. MUSCLE

MEATAL SKIN FLAP

DIGASTRIC MUSCLE

STERNO-CLEIDO-
MAST. MUSCLE

C

3.5 cm

1.5 cm   7.5 cm

MUSCULAR LAYER

SUBCUTANEOUS LAYER

Fig. **98 C**

**Mobilization of the occipital myosubcu-
taneous flap**

The retroauricular skin is separated from the subcutaneous soft tissues with a No. 20 blade, just
below the dermis. The initial musculoperiosteal incision (see Fig. 87 B) is extended posteriorly and inferiorly to the underlying bone using thermo-
cautery. The outlined myosubcutaneous flap has a
base of 3.5 cm, a length of 7.5 cm, and a width of
1.5 cm at the tip. The medial surface of the flap is
elevated from the bone using a mastoid raspatory.
The black arrows in the mastoid cavity show the insufficiently exteriorized retrofacial and retrolabyrinthine cells. A temporalis muscle flap is not used
because it would prevent sufficient superior exteriorization of the upper opening of the cavity.

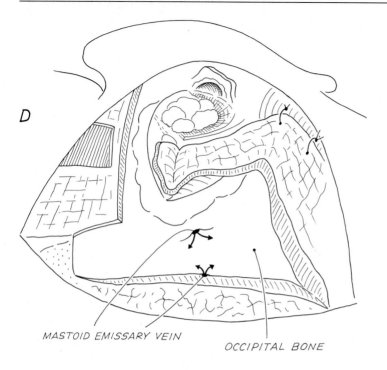

D

MASTOID EMISSARY VEIN

OCCIPITAL BONE

Fig. **98 D**

Obliteration of the posterior cavity with the occipital myosubcutaneous flap

The anteriorly transposed myosubcutaneous flap fills the retrofacial and retrolabyrinthine spaces behind the meatal skin flap. Catgut sutures keep the base of the flap in position over the digastric muscle and sigmoid sinus. Bleeding from mastoid emissary veins is stopped by drilling with a diamond burr without irrigation. Fibrin glue is used for further fixation of the flap to the bottom of the retrofacial and retrolabyrinthine spaces. Note that the tip of the flap does not include the temporalis muscle. Inclusion of the temporalis muscle in the flap would lead to necrosis due to insufficient blood supply.

The occipital myosubcutaneous flap is well vascularized by the occipital artery. Retraction may occur in time, but in a caudal and not a lateral direction as seen with the Palva flap. Trimming of superficial necrotic portions of the flap is performed as an office procedure with tympanoplasty scissors through the enlarged external canal (meatoplasty). Complete healing of the posterior obliterated cavity may require 2–3 months. During the first 4–6 weeks a Terracortril gauze is placed in the cavity and changed weekly. After this time, a cotton ball is placed in the meatus for protection. Antibiotic coverage (Bactrim, Augmentin) is continued for 10 days postoperatively.

4.3 Exteriorization of the Epitympanum

In poorly pneumatized temporal bones, the exenterated attic can be adequately exteriorized by bone removal. In highly pneumatized temporal bones, correct exteriorization of a deep supralabyrinthine space is impossible. In this case, obliteration with a free muscle graft is necessary.

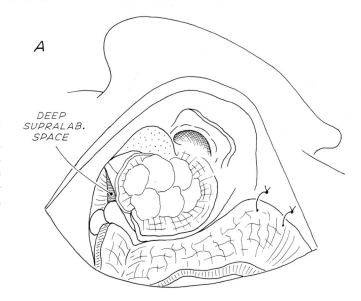

Fig. 99 A

Deep supralabyrinthine space

The occipital myosubcutaneous flap obliterates the retrofacial and retrolabyrinthine cells. Correct exteriorization of the supralabyrinthine recess is impossible because of the prominent tympanic facial nerve and bony ampulla of the lateral semicircular canal.

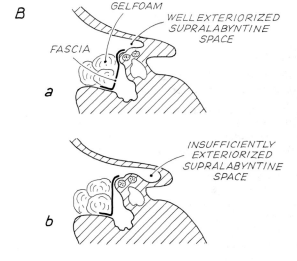

Fig. 99 B

Exteriorization of the supralabyrinthine recess

a: Sclerotic bone with adequate exteriorization.
b: Highly pneumatized bone with insufficient exteriorization.

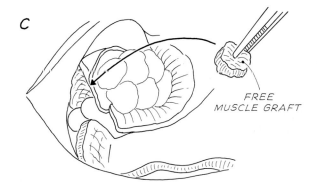

Fig. 99 C

Obliteration of a deep supralabyrinthine space

A free temporalis muscle graft is used to obliterate a deep supralabyrinthine recess.

5. Meatoplasty

Meatoplasty is systematically performed in open cavities regardless of the degree of mastoid pneumatization. The open cavity should have the shape of an inverted truncated cone. The bottom of the cavity involves both the cavum tympani and attic. Therefore, adequate shaping of the entrance implies widening the meatus. The meatoplasty is necessary for the correct exteriorization and self-cleansing property of an open cavity. This is true even after posterior obliteration with a myosubcutaneous flap. The meatoplasty is made as large as required by the shape of the bony cavity. Granulation tissue and the myosubcutaneous flap will provide a natural reduction in the size of the cavity entrance. Failure to perform meatoplasty in an open cavity will lead to a chronic secretion and to retention cholesteatoma because of inadequate exteriorization (see results, p. 195).

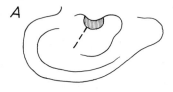

Fig. **100 A**

Conchal incision

The concha is incised with a No. 11 blade. The incision goes through the skin and cartilage and is directed posterosuperiorly toward the sinodural angle.

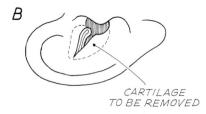

CARTILAGE
TO BE REMOVED

Fig. **100 B**

Removal of conchal cartilage

Sufficient cartilage (*broken line*) is removed on each side of the incision to allow introduction of the tip of the little finger into the open cavity. Note that the root of the anthelix is included in the resection to allow sufficient superior exteriorization of the cavity.

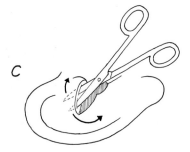

Fig. **100 C**

Elevation of skin from conchal cartilage

Curved tympanoplasty scissors are used to elevate the skin from the conchal cartilage.

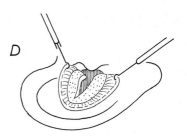

Fig. 100 D

Exposure of conchal cartilage

The mobilized skin is elevated with skin hooks, exposing the cartilage.

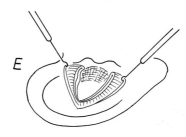

Fig. 100 E

Meatal entrance after excision of conchal cartilage

View of the meatal entrance after removal of the conchal cartilage with tympanoplasty scissors.

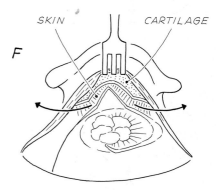

SKIN   CARTILAGE

Fig. 100 F

Inward rotation of conchal skin flaps

The auricle is rotated anteriorly, and the soft tissues medial to the conchal cartilage are mobilized with tympanoplasty scissors. Further resection is necessary if the skin flaps do not cover the edge of the remaining conchal cartilage. A free edge of cartilage may lead to perichondritis.

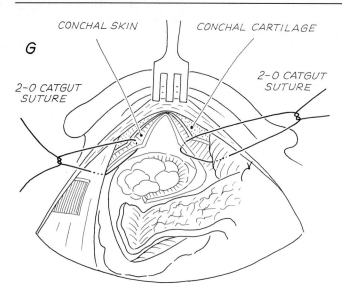

CONCHAL SKIN   CONCHAL CARTILAGE

G

2-0 CATGUT SUTURE

2-0 CATGUT SUTURE

Fig. **100 G**

Lateral fixation of conchal skin flaps

The conchal skin flaps are anchored with 2–0 Catgut sutures to the temporalis muscle (superiorly) and the mastoid soft tissues (inferiorly). The knots of the sutures are left loose and tightened only after posterior replacement of the pinna. If needed, one or two supplementary sutures are used to give the desired round shape to the meatal opening.

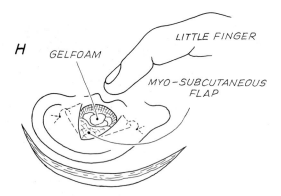

H   GELFOAM

LITTLE FINGER

MYO–SUBCUTANEOUS FLAP

Fig. **100 H**

Completed meatoplasty

The anchoring sutures of the conchal skin have been tightened. The Gelfoam packing (anteriorly) and the occipital myosubcutaneous flap (posteriorly) are visible through the enlarged meatal opening, which can easily accomodate the tip of the little finger.

6. Wound Closure and Packing

Fig. 101 A

Wound closure and packing

The retroauricular wound is closed in two layers using 2–0 Catgut and 3–0 Ethibond sutures. Gauze impregnated with Terracortril ointment is introduced over the Gelfoam.

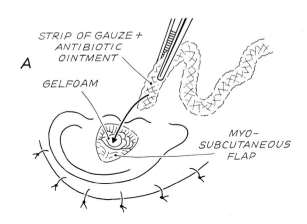

Fig. 101 B

Schematic view of the open cavity after packing

The anterior remnant of the tympanic membrane and the meatal skin are kept in place by Gelfoam soaked in Otosporin. A strip of gauze impregnated with Terracortril ointment fills the lateral portion of the cavity. A larger gauze is placed over the pinna and is kept in place with adhesive tape for further protection.

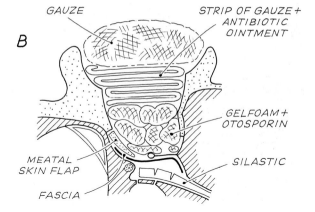

7. Results of Surgery for Cholesteatoma

7.1 Recurrent and Residual Cholesteatoma

The criteria for open or closed cavity in the management of cholesteatoma are given on p. 153 (choice of approach). Tables **16** and **17** show the 10-year follow-up results for 301 patients. In *children* (Table **16**) the rate of *residual cholesteatoma* was 25% in closed cavities (ICW) and 8% in open cavities (RMET). The rate of *recurrent* cholesteatoma was 13% in closed and 8% in open cavities. There is no statistical difference between the number of residual and recurrent cholesteatomas in closed and open cavities, regardless of the type of procedure performed. This lack of significance may be the result of the small number of patients available for late follow-up. The three failures in the open cavity group were related to insufficient exenteration of the supralabyrinthine recess, to inadequate lowering of the facial ridge, and to a narrow meatoplasty. These failures illustrate how important it is to perform the steps of an open mastoido-epitympanectomy correctly.

In *adults* (Table **17**), the rates of *residual* cholesteatoma were 8% for closed cavities (ICW) and 2% for open cavities (RMET). A recurrent cholesteatoma was found in 4% of the closed cavities and in none of the open cavities. The difference is statistically significant ($p < 0.05$) for both residual and recurrent cholesteatomas. This speaks in favor of the open cavity technique.

The comparison between the results of children and adults shows a significantly higher number of residual and recurrent cholesteatomas in the former for both open and closed cavities (38% and 12%, respectively in ICW, $p < 0.05$, and 16% vs. 2% in RMET, $p < 0.01$). The data shown in Tables **16** and **17** demonstrate that despite strict adherence to the listed criteria, it is possible to minimize but not to eliminate entirely the problem of residual or recurrent disease. The partial obliteration of the posterior cavity with the occipital myosubcutaneous flap has reduced the final size of an open cavity in such a dramatic way that our preference—with the exception of well-pneumatized and -ventilated mastoids—is constantly shifting toward the use of an open cavity technique for the management of cholesteatoma. The advantage of an open cavity is the minimal

Table **16**   Cholesteatoma: 10-year follow-up (children, n = 55)

Type of cavity	n	(%)	Residual cholest.		Recurrent cholest.		Residual + Recurrent	
ICW	16	(29)	4	(25)	2	(13)	6	(38)
RMET	39	(71)	3	(8)	3	(8)	6	(16)
Total	55	(100)	7	(13)	5	(9)	12	(22)

Table **17**   Cholesteatoma: 10-year follow-up (adults, n = 246)

Type of cavity	n	(%)	Residual cholest.		Recurrent cholest.		Residual + Recurrent	
ICW	134	(54)	11	(8)	5	(4)	16	(12)
RMET	112	(46)	2	(2)	–	–	2	(2)
Total	246	(100)	13	(5)	5	(2)	18	(7)

Table **18**   RMET for cholesteatoma: condition of operative cavity 10 years postop. (children n = 55; adults n = 246)

Type of cavity	Children				Adults			
	Dry		Wet		Dry		Wet	
	n	(%)	n	(%)	n	(%)	n	(%)
ICW	15/16	(94)	1/16	(6)	129/134	(96)	5/134	(4)
RMET	36/39	(92)	3/39	(8)	106/112	(95)	6/112	(5)

risk of residual and recurrent disease. Furthermore, in an open MET, persisting or recurring cholesteatoma is limited to the cavum tympani (mainly oval and round window niches, sinus tympani) where it can more readily be detected by clinical inspection without the necessity of second-look surgery.

7.2 Postoperative Cavity Problems

Postoperative cavity problems are frequently mentioned as a disadvantage of open cavity procedures. Table **18** shows the conditions of the operative cavity in 301 patients who underwent surgery because of a cholesteatoma. There is no statistical difference between the rate of dry (and self-cleansing) open and closed cavities (94% vs. 92% in children, 96% vs. 95% in adults). These figures demonstrate that a correctly performed open cavity does not represent an inconvenience to the patients and invalidate the main objection to open cavity surgery. The minimal number of cavity problems of an open MET has to be related to the use of the occipital myosubcutaneous flap for posterior cavity obliteration. Measurements of the cavity volume have shown that the average size of an obliterated open cavity is only twice the size of a normal external canal (1.5 ml vs. 0.7 ml).

7.3 Revision Surgery in Open Cavity

Revision surgery of 79 consecutive patients with draining radical mastoidectomy cavities

has shown that the reason for the failure was not inherent to the type of surgery but to the quality of its execution.

The main causes for failure were:
1. Incomplete exenteration of cellular tracts (55/79 = 70% of the cases, see Fig. **102**, see p. 196)
2. Inadequate exteriorization of the cavity (73/79 = 92% of the cases, see Fig. **103**, see p. 196)
3. Inadequate ventilation owing to absent or insufficient meatoplasty (41/73 = 56% of the cases)

Incomplete exenteration of retrofacial and retrolabyrinthine cells was also due to the anterior position of the retroauricular incision performed in the postauricular sulcus in most instances. Radical exenteration of the supralabyrinthine cells requires a good knowledge of the location of the superior semicircular canal and of the labyrinthine segment of the facial nerve.

The inadequate exteriorization of the cavity was mainly related to the failure to remove bone over the middle cranial fossa dura, the sigmoid sinus, the mastoid segment of the facial nerve, and in the region of the mastoid tip. The elimination of unnecessarily high and overhanging bony walls leads to a considerable reduction of the size of the cavity.

The meatoplasty was inadequate in 41/73 (56%) of the cases. The enlargement of the meatus is an integral part of shaping an open cavity in the form of an inverted truncated cone. Even the most perfectly executed mastoido-epitympanectomy will fail if its ventilation is not secured by adequate meatoplasty.

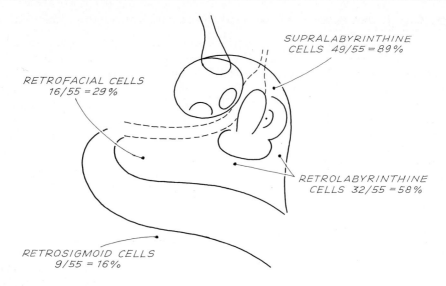

Fig. **102**

Incomplete exenteration of cellular tracts in open cavity

Localization of residual cellular tracts in 55/79 (70%) of draining radical mastoidectomies.

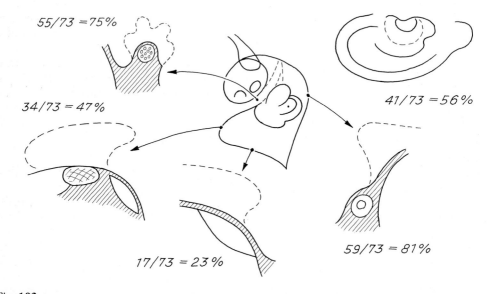

Fig. **103**

Inadequate exteriorization of open cavity

The middle fossa dura, the sigmoid sinus, the mastoid tip, and the facial ridge were inadequately removed in 73/79 (92%) of the draining radical mastoidectomies.

8. Rules and Hints

- The surgical treatment of acquired cholesteatoma has to be tailored to the needs of the individual patient, depending upon the skill, experience, and clinical judgement of the surgeon.
- Do not use a single surgical procedure, but a system of operations.
- Opening the cholesteatoma sac to evacuate its contents improves visualization without increasing the risk of residual cholesteatoma.
- By removing the contents of a cholesteatoma sac, defects of the labyrinthine bone (fistula) can be identified without elevating the matrix.
- Always expect a fistula in cholesteatoma, even if the patient does not have vertigo.
- The degree of pneumatization will influence the decision to perform an open or closed cavity.
- The best indication of long-term eustachian tube function is the extent of temporal bone pneumatization.
- Secondary acquired cholesteatoma is *not* a radiologic diagnosis.

Closed Cavity

- Perform an open cavity when complete removal of the matrix is not possible beyond doubt.
- Systematic epitympanectomy includes removal of the incus, malleus head, and tensor chorda fold.
- Posterior tympanotomy may be a necessary adjunct of epitympanectomy.
- Use septal or tragal cartilage to reinforce the posterosuperior meatal wall and posterosuperior quadrant of the new drum.
- Use thick Silastic or Gelfilm sheeting whenever staging is necessary.
- Acute viral mastoiditis is more dangerous to the inner ear than acute suppurative mastoiditis.
- Adequate drainage of the oval and round window in acute viral mastoiditis may require posterior tympanotomy when granulation tissue prevents adequate drainage through a ventilating tube placed in the drum.
- Do not lower the bony posterior entrance of the ear canal when performing canalplasty or antrotomy.
- Canalplasty should be performed first to define the anterior limit of the mastoidectomy.
- Leave the preserved canal wall as thick as possible (particularly the area close to the tympanic membrane) to prevent resorption.
- When removing the matrix from the oval window using the combined approach, be aware of a possible dehiscent facial nerve.
- EMG monitoring of facial muscles prevents lesion of the facial nerve when performing posterior tympanotomy and removing obscure disease from the oval and round windows.
- Transmastoid drainage is helpful in supporting ventilation and cleansing of the middle ear in the postoperative period, particularly when eustachian tube function is marginal.
- Stage ossicular reconstruction whenever the malleus handle is missing (exception: tympanoplasty type III).
- The sheeting used in staged surgery should extend into the eustachian tube orifice (tubotympanic sheeting).

Open Cavity

- A draining open cavity is not the fault of the surgery but of the surgeon.
- The more bone you remove, the smaller the surgical cavity.
- Do not leave bony overhangs.
- Skeletonize the middle cranial fossa dura for adequate superior exteriorization of the open cavity.
- Remove bone over and behind the sigmoid sinus for adequate reduction of the cavity volume.
- Remove the mastoid tip to reduce the cavity volume.

- Provide adequate ventilation of the cavity with meatoplasty.
- Exenterated cellular tracts are not necessarily adequately exteriorized.
- The principle of the "inverted truncated cone" should not only apply to the main cavity but to all minor exenterated spaces as well.
- Spaces that cannot be adequately exteriorized should be obliterated.
- Wide lateral removal of bone results in a considerable reduction in the volume of the open cavity.
- The epitympanum should be managed as radically as the mastoid (radical epitympanectomy).
- Exteriorization of the attic in the open cavity does not affect the functional results of surgery.
- In the presence of a mobile, intact stapes, type III tympanoplasty may be performed in one stage.
- Staged surgery should be used in the footplate only situation (exception: tympanoplasty type IV).

- A type IV tympanoplasty may be performed in cases of marginal eustachian tube function and shallow middle ear cavity.
- The use of the occipital myosubcutaneous flap has nearly eliminated the necessity of reconstructing an open cavity.
- The final size of an open cavity is determined by the natural formation of granulations in the presence of an adequate meatoplasty in conjunction with the use of an occipital myosubcutaneous flap.
- Application of a skin graft to the open cavity would prevent the natural volume reduction of the cavity produced by granulation during the healing process.
- Preservation of the skin at the anterior tympanomeatal angle is important for the vibratory properties of the neotympanum.
- Reepithelization of the open cavity proceeds from the meatal skin flap, the skin remnant of the anterior tympanomeatal angle, and the conchal skin flaps.

Chapter 6
Special Applications of Mastoidectomy

1. Reconstruction of Open Cavity

1.1 General Concepts

The indication for the reconstruction of a properly performed open cavity is rarely given because the wide lateral removal of bone and the posterior obliteration of the cavity with occipital myosubcutaneous flap will produce small cavities with an average volume of 1.5 ml.

The reconstruction of an open cavity may be associated with

– a ventilated mastoid (Figs. **104 A, B**) or
– an obliterated mastoid (Fig. **104 C**).

The principles of the various types of reconstruction are shown in the following figures. Reconstruction of a ventilated mastoid is seldom performed because, in the long term, the eustachian tube problems that have created the initial disease often manifest themselves again.

1.2 Surgical Technique

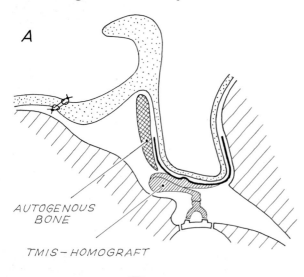

A

AUTOGENOUS
BONE

TMIS – HOMOGRAFT

Fig. **104 A**

Reconstruction of open cavity with ventilated mastoid, using autogenous bone and drum, ossicles homograft

Autogenous bone from the retroauricular region and from the temporal squama (see Fig. 55 A–F) is used to reconstruct the posterior wall in association with homograft ossicles. This type of reconstruction has been disappointing in the long term because of recurrent disease induced by defective ventilation in the attic and mastoid with poor functional results.

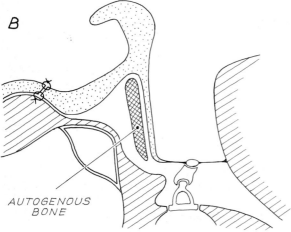

B

AUTOGENOUS
BONE

Fig. **104 B**

Reconstruction of open cavity with ventilated mastoid, using autogenous bone and fascia

The attempt to associate the advantage of epitympanectomy (ossicular bypass of the attic) when reconstructing an open cavity with a ventilated mastoid has also proven unsuccessful in the long term. It is probably too optimistic to expect complete re-epithelization of a ventilated attic and mastoid from a minimal mucosal lining confined to the protympanum.

Fig. **104 C**

Reconstruction of open cavity with an obliterated mastoid

Obliteration of the mastoid with auto-genous bone paste (bone dust mixed with fibrin glue) has been more successful than attempts to reventilate the mastoid and attic. However, partial breakdown of the reconstructed meatal wall may occur in time, producing irregularities that limit the self-cleansing property of the cavity. This change in the shape of the cavity may also induce the danger of retention cholesteatoma. This is why, before recon-struction, the bony cavity should be shaped as an open mastoido-epitym-panectomy. This implies the extensive re-moval of lateral tympanomastoid bone and the adequate meatoplasty. At present we prefer to fill the mastoid with an occipi-tal myosubcutaneous flap (as described on pp. 187–188, Fig. 98 C–D) and to incor-porate the attic in the open cavity.

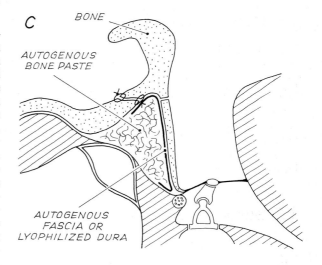

2. Cochlear Implant

Surgical Technique

The described surgical steps relate to the im-plantation of a Nucleus 22 channel Cochlear Implant.*

The operation is carried out under general anesthesia.

Surgical Highlights

- L-shaped retroauricular incision for skin flap
- Inverted L-shaped incision for musculo-periosteal flap

- Circular bed for receiver/stimulator package drilled behind the sinodural angle
- Partial mastoidectomy
- Retrograde exposure of mastoid seg-ment of fallopian canal
- Posterior tympanotomy with exposure of round window niche
- Formation of mastoid groove for the electrode lead
- Fixation of receiver/stimulator package in its bony bed
- Introduction of electrode array into the basal turn of the cochlea
- Fixation of electrode lead in its bony groove
- Wound closure in layers

---

* Cochlear PTY, Ltd., 1 Woodcock Place, Lane Cave 2066, Sydney, Australia

Surgical Steps

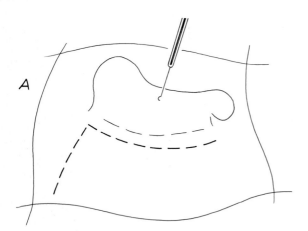

Fig. **105 A**

Skin incision

The L-shaped retroauricular skin incision; the longer limb is close to the retroauricular sulcus and the shorter limb is along the temporal line.

Fig. **105 B**

Musculoperiosteal flap

A reverse L-shaped incision is used for the musculoperiosteal flap, which is based superiorly in contrast to the skin flap.

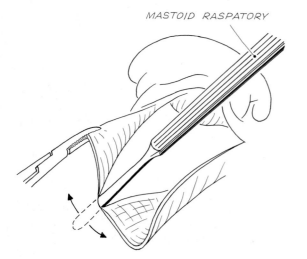

Fig. **105 C**

Elevation of parietosquamous periosteum

The periosteum is widely elevated from the bone posterosuperiorly to stabilize the flange of the implanted receiver/stimulator package.

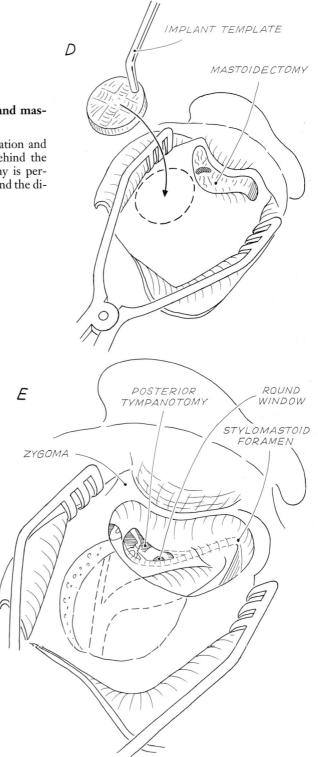

Fig. **105 D**

Bed for receiver/stimulator package and mastoidectomy

A template is used to determine the location and size of the circular bed to be drilled behind the sinodural angle. A partial mastoidectomy is performed, skeletonizing the sigmoid sinus and the digastric muscle.

Fig. **105 E**

Posterior tympanotomy

The circular bed for the receiver/stimulator package is centered on the confluence of the superior petrosal and sigmoid sinuses. The stylomastoid foramen is identified along the digastric ridge and stylomastoid periosteum. The lateral semicircular canal and the short process of the incus are exposed. The mastoid segment of the facial nerve is skeletonized to the level of the posterior semicircular canal. The posterior tympanotomy is carried out between the exposed pyramidal segment of the facial nerve and the chorda tympani. Knowledge of the location of the facial nerve accelerates this step and allows for wide exposure of the round window niche (see also Fig. 80 M). EMG monitoring of the facial muscles (NIM-2) is helpful for this preparation.

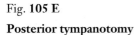

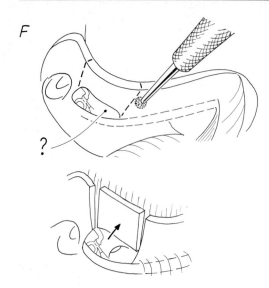

Fig. 105 F

Temporary anterior dislocation of posterior canal wall for exposure of the round window niche

The round window niche may not be sufficiently exposed because of a prominent facial nerve. A segment of the posterior canal wall is mobilized with a diamond burr. The mobilized bony segment is displaced anteriorly for adequate exposure of the round window niche.

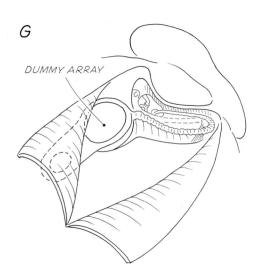

Fig. 105 G

Introduction of cochlear implant

The final position of the cochlear implant is tested with a dummy array, which includes the electrode lead. In this way, the position of the bony groove in the mastoid for the electrode lead is determined.

Fig. 105 H

Mastoid groove for electrode fixation

A bony groove is drilled along the inner surface of the mastoid tip and posterior canal wall to stabilize the electrode. This avoids the need for the complicated Dacron mesh ties described in the literature. The chorda tympani may have to be sacrificed in narrow mastoids.

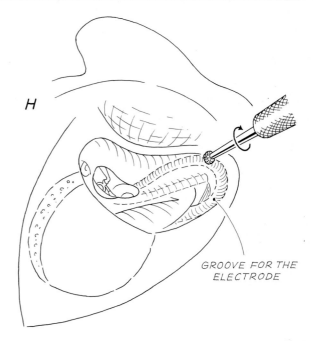

GROOVE FOR THE
ELECTRODE

Fig. 105 I

Cochleostomy

The superior rim of the round window niche is removed until the lumen of the basal turn is exposed. High-resolution CT scans are required to determine the amount of ossification present in this part of the inner ear. The lumen of the basal turn of the cochlea was reached in 24 out of 25 ears operated on. In one instance, the scala tympani of the basal turn was completely ossified, and the electrode had to be placed in the scala vestibuli following removal of the stapes.

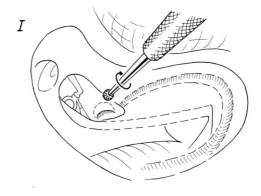

Fig. 105 J

Introduction of the electrodes in the scala tympani

The tip of the electrode array is placed with watchmaker forceps in the 1–2-mm opening drilled in the basal turn. The electrodes are then advanced inside the scala tympani with a special claw for electrode insertion, if no resistance is felt. The insertion is continued until the electrode array is completely within the cochlea.

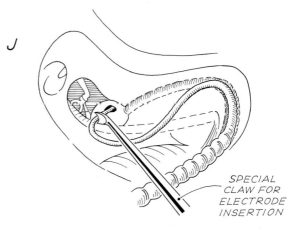

SPECIAL
CLAW FOR
ELECTRODE
INSERTION

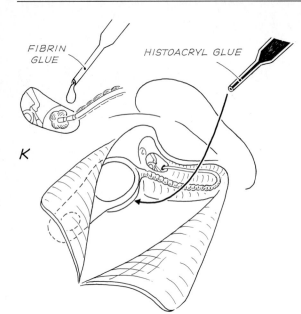

FIBRIN GLUE

HISTOACRYL GLUE

K

Fig. **105 K**

Electrode array and receiver/stimulator package in position

The round window niche is sealed with connective tissue and fibrin glue. Histoacryl glue*, or, more recently, ionomer bone cement is used for fixation of the electrode lead and of the receiver/stimulator package in its mastoid bed.

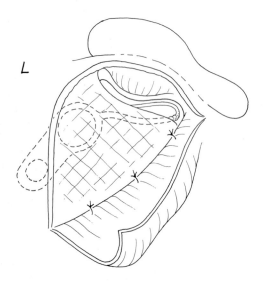

L

Fig. **105 L**

Wound closure

The superiorly based musculoperiosteal flap is repositioned, completely covering the implant.

* B. Braun AG, 34212 Melsungen, Germany

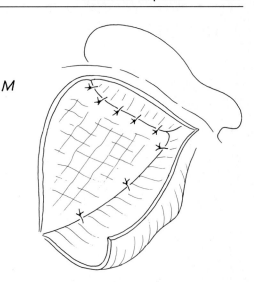

M

Fig. **105 M**

Wound closure (cont.)

2–0 Dexon sutures fix the musculoperiosteal flap to the surrounding soft tissues. The mastoid cavity is completely covered by the anterior edge of the musculoperiosteal flap.

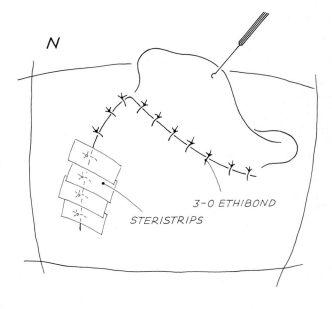

N

Fig. **105 N**

Wound closure (cont.)

The skin incision is closed with 3–0 Ethibond sutures supplemented by Steristrips. The sutures are left in place for 10 days. The patient receives antibiotic coverage (Bactrim or Augmentin) for 5 days.

3. Results

3.1 Reconstruction of Open Cavity

The results of reconstruction of an open cavity with ventilated mastoid (see Figs. **104 A, B**) have been disappointing at the long term. The defective function of the eustachian tube has led to recurrent disease and poor functional results. It is probably too optimistic to expect extensive reepithelization of middle ear and mastoid from a minimal residual lining of mucosa confined to the protympanum. Obliteration of the mastoid has been more successful than attempts to reventilate the mastoid. However, partial breakdown of the reconstructed meatal wall is always possible. This may compromise the adequate exteriorization and reduce the self-cleansing property of the reconstructed cavity.

Our preference, to date, goes to obliteration of the mastoid with an occipital myosubcutaneous flap (see Fig. 98 C–D). The attic is incorporated into the external auditory canal. The bony cavity is shaped as in an open mastoido-epitympanectomy with extensive lateral removal of bone. The meatoplasty is carried out as if the mastoid would not be obliterated. This avoids cavity problems in case of partial or total breakdown of the reconstructed canal wall.

3.2 Cochlear Implant

In the past 10 years, 28 Nucleus devices have been implanted in 21 adults and 7 children. The use of overlapping, reverse-pedicled skin and musculoperiosteal flaps has avoided any immediate or delayed complication of wound healing. Two revision operations were necessary because of technical defects of the implant. These were related to the electronics within the receiver/stimulator package. No adverse effects of the methacrylate glue (Histoacryl) used for fixation of the electrode lead and receiver/stimulator package was observed. The duration of the implantation procedure was, on average, 55 minutes.

The position and depth of the bony bed for the implant was found adequate in all instances. A more posterior and superior bed would carry the risk of an insufficient thickness of the underlying bone with possible CSF leak, particularly in children. Recently, we had to revise a child with a Nucleus implant carried out successfully elsewhere. The receiver/stimulator package had been implanted above the temporal line. The patient developed three spells of meningitis after surgery. The bed for the implant was in communication with a granulation of Pacchioni situated within the very tiny diploë of the bone.

4. Rules and Hints

Reconstructed Cavity

- Reconstruction of an open cavity with ventilated mastoid presupposes perfect eustachian tube function.
- Insufficient eustachian tube function is the most frequent cause of disease requiring an open cavity.
- Atrophy or breakdown of a reconstructed canal wall compromises the adequate shape of the external canal. This may cause chronic drainage and retention cholesteatoma.
- If an occipital myosubcutaneous flap is used to reconstruct the mastoid, shape the bony cavity and the meatoplasty as for an open MET.
- An adequate meatoplasty allows for natural adaptation of the volume of the new external auditory canal. This process may require 4–6 weeks.
- Don't ask too much from the limited mucosal lining of an open cavity undergoing reconstruction.
- Resurfacing the mesotympanum and hypotympanum with a new mucosal lining is

sufficient for successful, staged functional surgery.

- An adequately formed open cavity gives better results than a reconstructed closed cavity if the function of the eustachian tube is defective.
- At the long term, a reconstructed open cavity with ventilated mastoid requires reconversion into its original state in the majority of cases because of insufficient eustachian tube function.

Cochlear Implant

- The use of overlapping skin and musculoperiosteal flaps avoids problems of wound healing.
- Drilling the bed for the receiver/stimulator package should take place behind the sinodural angle.
- The bony bed for the implant should be drilled *before* the mastoidectomy to secure sufficient anterior support by bone.
- Skeletonization of the mastoid segment of the fallopian canal starting from the sty-

lomastoid foramen facilitates the adequate exposure of the round window niche through a posterior tympanotomy.

- Drilling of a mastoid groove for fixation of the electrode lead avoids the need for complicated Dacron mesh ties.
- If the round window niche is difficult to see because of a narrow space between tympanic margin and facial nerve, the cochleostomy may be performed by direct drilling over the posterior edge of the promontory.
- Elevation of the parietosquamous periosteum gives sufficient fixation for the flange of the receiver/stimulator package.
- The repositioned musculoperiosteal flap covers the complete implant and provides additional stabilization for it.
- Histoacryl glue or Ionocement may be used for extra fixation of the receiver/stimulator package in its bony bed.
- After the electrode array has been inserted, the cochleostomy is best closed with a free muscle graft and fibrin glue.

Chapter 7
Stapes Surgery

General Considerations

1. Stapedotomy versus Stapedectomy

In our department, the limited central perforation of the footplate (*stapedotomy*) has replaced the partial (small *fenestra*) or total removal of the stapes footplate (*stapedectomy*) since 1978 for reasons illustrated in Figs. **106 A, B, C.**

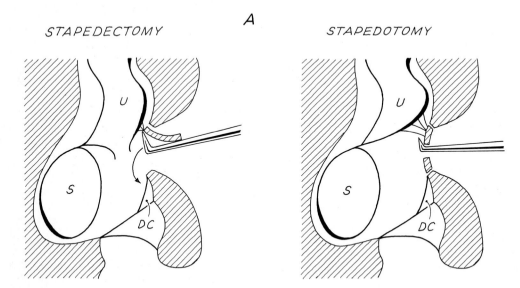

A

Fig. **106 A**

Less risk of inner ear damage in stapedotomy

A 0.4-mm stapedotomy carries less risk of inner ear damage than a total or subtotal stapedectomy. Correct total removal of the footplate may induce a sensorineural hearing loss and vertigo because of the unavoidable damage of the utricle when superior fibrous adhesions are present in the vestibule. Fibrous adhesions between the superior footplate and the utricle were found in two-thirds of the normal temporal bones of our histological collection.

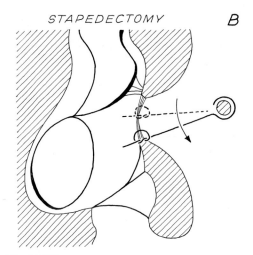

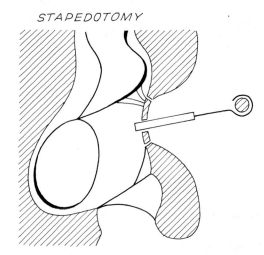

Fig. 106 B

Less probability of prosthesis migration after stapedotomy

A limited perforation through the footplate (stapedotomy) prevents lateral displacement of the prosthesis due to traction of postoperative scar-ring. A wire connective-tissue prosthesis used with stapedectomy can migrate toward the inferior or superior edge of the oval window. This has been found to induce conductive or even sensorineural hearing loss and vertigo (lesion of the endolymphatic duct and/or utricle)

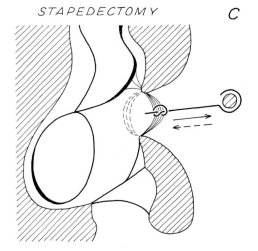

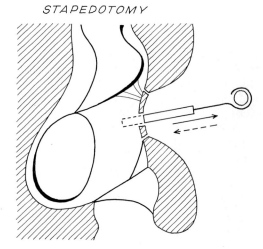

Fig. 106 C

No lateral displacement of the oval window membrane in stapedotomy

The membrane, which covers the open oval window after stapedectomy, may be displaced laterally by (1) an increase in perilymphatic pressure, (2) scar retraction, particularly with a wire connective tissue prosthesis that is too short, or (3) by movements of the incus following sneezing or rapid changes in middle ear pressure. Revision surgery shows that the lateral displacement of the oval win-dow membrane can cause lateralization of the properly sized prosthesis with incus erosion. It is also possible that incus movements due to barotrauma (flying, crossing mountains by car) may cause a sudden hearing loss years after a successful stapedectomy. This complication is less likely to occur after stapedotomy since, in the latter case, the prosthesis may be pulled out from the stapedotomy opening without causing adverse effects to the inner ear.

Specific Surgical Techniques

1. Stapedotomy

Surgical Technique

The surgical steps of stapedotomy are demonstrated for otosclerosis since this condition is the most common indication for the procedure. The use of a 0.4-mm Teflon Platinum Piston (TPP) has allowed reversal of the classic steps of stapes surgery. The stapedotomy opening as well as the introduction and fixation of the TPP, is done *before* division of the incudostapedial joint and *before* removal of the stapes arch. The reversal of the classic steps of stapes surgery permits formation of a central stapedotomy opening without mobilization or fracture of the footplate. Furthermore, the prosthesis loop can be better attached to the incus when the incus remains stabilized by the intact incudostapedial joint. This avoids the danger of incus luxation or excessive displacement of the prosthesis into the vestibule while crimping. The use of a 0.4-mm piston is essential to reverse systematically the classic steps of stapes surgery. The limited space between the stapes arch and facial nerve prevents the consistent use of larger (0.6-mm or 0.8-mm) pistons.

Surgical Highlights

- Local anesthesia
- Endaural skin incision
- Elevation of tympanomeatal flap
- Exposure of oval window
- Trimming and storage of a 0.4-mm TPP on the special cutting block
- Stapedotomy with manual perforators
- Introduction and fixation of TPP with intact incudostapedial joint and stapes arch
- Division of stapes arch with prosthesis in place using crurotomy scissors.
- Sealing of stapedotomy opening with connective tissue, venous blood, and fibrin glue
- Packing with Gelfoam
- Closure of endaural incision

Surgical Steps

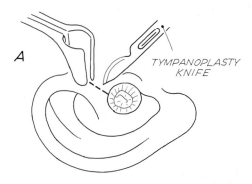

A

TYMPANOPLASTY KNIFE

Fig. **107 A**

Endaural skin incision

A helicotragal skin incision is carried out using a No. 15 blade while enlarging the external canal with a nasal speculum.

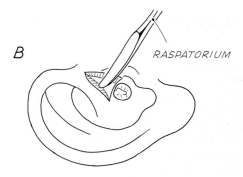

B

RASPATORIUM

Fig. **107 B**

Widening of external auditory canal

An endaural raspatory is used to separate the soft tissues from the underlying bone at the superior edge of the external auditory canal.

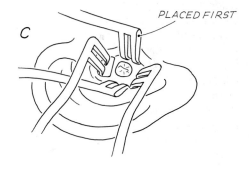

PLACED FIRST

C

Fig. **107 C**

Widening of external auditory canal (cont.)

Two endaural retractors are placed perpendicular to each other over the entrance of the external auditory canal to give the necessary exposure.

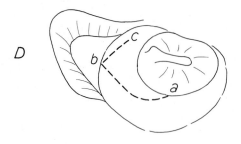

Fig. **107 D**

Tympanomeatal flap

The triangular tympanomeatal flap has a posterior limb (*a – b*) that begins at 8 o'clock, ascending spirally from the tympanic annulus to the lateral edge of the external auditory canal. The anterior limb of the tympanomeatal incision (**b – c**) descends from the lateral opening of the external canal along the tympanosquamous suture toward the lateral process of the malleus. The intrameatal incisions are carried out with a rounded scalpel handle, carrying a No. 11 blade.

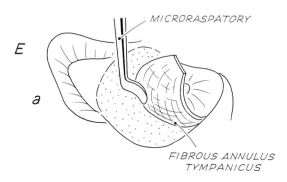

MICRORASPATORY

FIBROUS ANNULUS
TYMPANICUS

Fig. 107 E

Tympanomeatal flap (cont.)

a: The tympanomeatal flap is elevated from the underlying bone with the universal microraspatory.

b: The most important landmark in this step is the posterior tympanic spine (posterior end of the incisura tympanica Rivini).

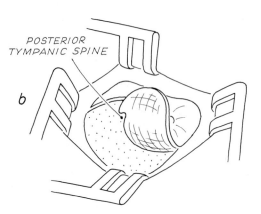

POSTERIOR
TYMPANIC SPINE

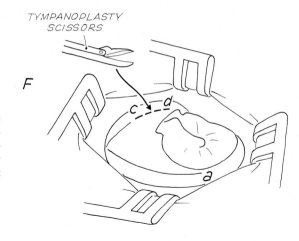

Fig. **107 F**

Tympanomeatal flap (cont.)

After exposure of the posterior tympanic spine, the anterior limb of the tympanomeatal incision is extended with tympanoplasty microscissors toward the anterior spine (c–d), remaining above the short process of the malleus.

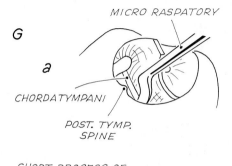

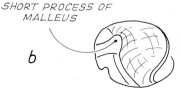

Fig. **107 G**

Tympanomeatal flap (cont.)

a: The elevation of the tympanic annulus from the tympanic sulcus begins at the posterior tympanic spine, using a universal microraspatory.

b: The chorda tympani is left attached to the retracted drum. The pars flaccida of the tympanic membrane is elevated with the universal microraspatory over the neck and short process of the malleus. A cartilagenous apophysis may be found over the lateral process of the malleus. This cartilage is elevated with the tympanomeatal flap. Exposure of the short process of the malleus keeps the tympanomeatal flap away and allows early determination of the mobility of this ossicle. Gelfoam soaked in 1% lidocaine solution is placed in the exposed middle ear cavity for 2 minutes if pain is experienced by the patient while the tympanomeatal flap is being elevated.

A

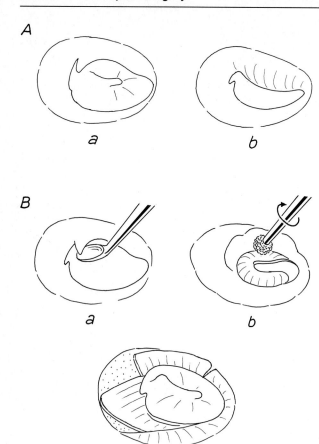

a

b

B

a

b

c

Fig. **108 A**

Canalplasty

Correct elevation of the tympanomeatal flap implies good visualization of the lateral process of the malleus. A prominent tympanosquamous
spine (**a**) or a prominent anterior wall
of the external canal (**b**) may prevent
adequate visualization.

Fig. **108 B**

Canalplasty (cont.)

The large end of a curette (**a**) or a diamond burr (**b**) is used to enlarge the external canal until the lateral process of
the malleus becomes visible. Using
the burr requires irrigation, which can
lead to contamination of the middle
ear. Therefore, canalplasty should be
carried out before elevating the tympanic annulus from the sulcus.

c: Correct exposure of the malleus following canalplasty.

Fig. 109 A

Exposure of the oval window

After elevation of the tympanomeatal flap, the bone covering the oval window niche is removed with the small end of a sharp curette. Care is taken to avoid trauma to the chorda tympani.

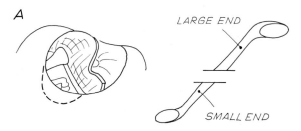

Fig. 109 B

Exposure of the oval window (cont.)

The rotational movements of the sharp curette are directed from medial to lateral when exposing the oval window. Bone fragments should be continuously removed to avoid inadvertent luxation of the incus by pushing them medially with the curette.

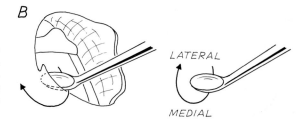

Fig. 109 C

Exposure of the oval window (cont.)

The correct exposure of the oval window is obtained when the short process of the malleus, the tympanic segment of the facial nerve, and the pyramidal process are visible. Visualization of these three landmarks is essential for correct execution of the further steps of surgery.

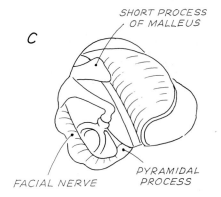

Fig. 109 D

Mobilization of the chorda tympani

At times the chorda tympani runs within the bony posterior canal wall, preventing correct exposure of the oval window (a). If this is the case, the bone covering the chorda has to be removed using the small end of a sharp curette (b) or with the universal microraspatory (c). The chorda tympani should be preserved whenever possible. However, if mobilization is impossible without lesion, the chorda is cut with tympanoplasty microscissors.

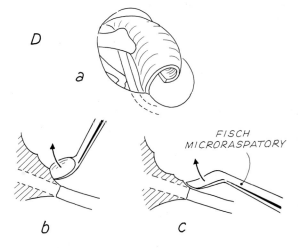

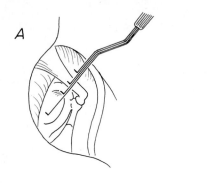

A

Fig. 110 A

Determination of prosthesis length

A malleable measuring rod is used to determine the distance between the footplate and the lateral surface of the incus (average length 4.7 mm); 0.5 mm are added to account for the protrusion of the prosthesis into the vestibule. The average total length of the prosthesis is, therefore, 5.2 mm. Manipulations of the mucosa of the oval window may cause pain. In this case, a Gelfoam pledget soaked in 1% lidocaine is placed in the oval window for 2 minutes.

B

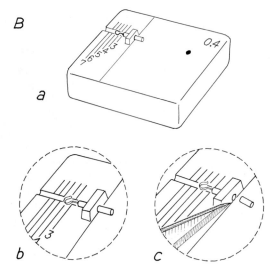

Fig. 110 B

Trimming the prosthesis

A special cutting block has been developed so that only one size prosthesis, a Teflon platinum band piston (TPP), 7 mm long, 0.4 mm diameter, is stocked. The prosthesis is trimmed on the cutting block (**a**). The prosthesis is placed on a groove of the cutting block and advanced with watchmaker forceps through the perforated bridge until the desired length is reached (**b**). The excess of the Teflon piston is cut away using a No. 11 blade (**c**).

C

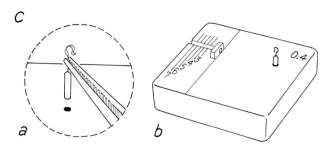

Fig. 110 C

Storage of prosthesis

The trimmed prosthesis is grasped with watchmaker forceps and placed in the 0.4-mm hole of the cutting block for later use.

Fig. 111 A

Safe area for stapedotomy

Measurements* made in normal and otosclerotic bones of our temporal bone collection* have shown that the saccule and utricle are more than 1 mm below the inferior central two-thirds of the stapes footplate. This is, therefore, the safest place for the stapedotomy opening.

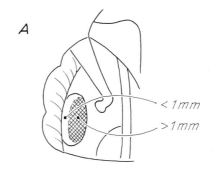

Fig. 111 B

Perforation of the footplate

A set of four manual perforators (0.3-, 0.4-, 0.5-, and 0.6-mm diameter) is used to make the stapedotomy opening in the footplate. The perforators are rotated back and forth between the thumb and index finger of the right hand. The tip of each perforator is only partially introduced into the vestibule. This is why the 0.6-mm diameter perforator produces an opening that is only slightly larger than 0.4 mm. The pressure applied to the perforator tip is minimal. The actual work is carried out with the perforator's shoulder.

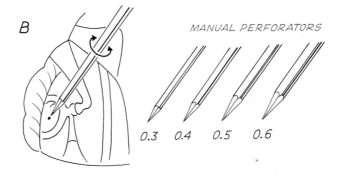

Fig. 111 C

Perforation of the footplate (cont.)

The correct size of the stapedotomy opening is confirmed with a malleable 0.4-mm measuring caliper. The stapedotomy opening should allow free movement of the tip of the caliper rod. An opening that is too narrow will hamper the proper free movements of the piston, which may lie at an oblique angle to the footplate.

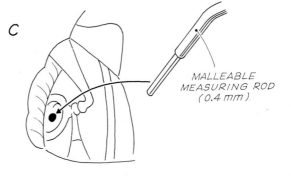

---

* Pauw, B., Pollak, A., Fisch, U. Annals: Otol Rhinol Laryngol 1991; 12: 960–970.

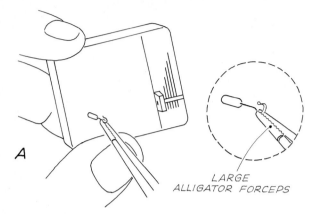

A

LARGE
ALLIGATOR FORCEPS

Fig. 112 A

Introduction of the prosthesis

The TPP is picked up from the cutting block with a large alligator forceps. The cutting block is held such that the alligator forceps is guided by the left thumb. Picking up the prosthesis at the proper angle is essential for correct placement.

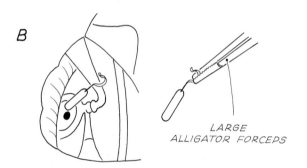

B

LARGE
ALLIGATOR FORCEPS

Fig. 112 B

Introduction of the prosthesis (cont.)

The TPP is first placed over the stapes footplate. The length is correct if the loop of the prosthesis lies 0.5 mm lateral to the incus. A prosthesis that is too long is replaced on the cutting for further trimming. A prosthesis that is too short is discarded and substituted with a new one.

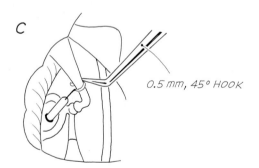

C

0.5 mm, 45° HOOK

Fig. 112 C

Introduction of the prosthesis (cont.)

After confirmation of its correct size, the prosthesis is moved over the stapedotomy opening and advanced into the vestibule with a 0.5-mm, 45° hook.

Fig. 112 D

Fixation of prosthesis to incus

The prosthesis loop is crimped over the incus with a large alligator forceps. This step is performed while the incudostapedial joint is still intact. This is not the case in conventional stapedectomy, where the stapes arch is removed before the prosthesis is placed. Reversal of the conventional stapedectomy steps is possible in 95% of the cases if a 0.4-mm piston is used. The space between the stapes arch and facial nerve is too narrow for larger (0.6-mm or 0.8-mm) pistons. The intact incudostapedial joint is the best guarantee against undue mobilization or fracture of the footplate. These invariably occur when the arch is broken off first. A further advantage of reversing the stapedotomy steps is that adaptation of the prosthesis loop to the incus is permitted without the danger of excessive protrusion of the piston in the vestibule or of incus luxation when crimping.

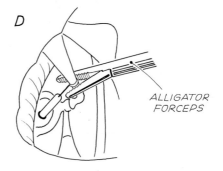

ALLIGATOR FORCEPS

Fig. 112 E

Prosthesis in place

The prosthesis is firmly attached to the incus. Proper adaptation requires perfect conformation of the platinum band to the incus. The piston protrudes 0.5 mm into the vestibule.

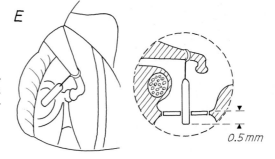

0.5 mm

A

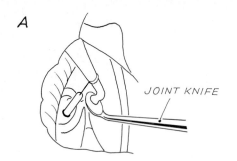

JOINT KNIFE

Fig. 113 A

Removal of stapes arch

The incudostapedial joint is separated with a joint knife. The mobility of the malleus and incus may be fully appreciated only after this step. If there is doubt, the incudostapedial joint may be separated before the prosthesis is introduced. This allows better evaluation of the mobility of the ossicles without destabilization of the incus.

B

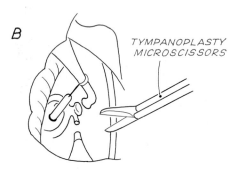

TYMPANOPLASTY
MICROSCISSORS

Fig. 113 B

Removal of stapes arch (cont.)

The stapedial tendon is cut with tympanoplasty microscissors.

C

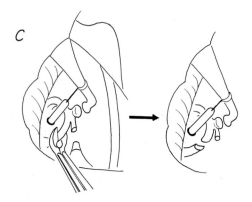

Fig. 113 C

Removal of stapes arch (cont.)

The posterior crus is cut with left crurotomy scissors. Right crurotomy scissors are used for the left ear. Exposure of the pyramidal process is necessary to provide sufficient space for the crurotomy.

Fig. 113 D

Removal of stapes arch (cont.)

a: The anterior crus is crushed at the level of the footplate with a 2.5-mm, 45° hook introduced between the incus and malleus handle.

b: A downward rotational movement is performed when the tip of the hook has reached the base of the anterior crus. In this way, the crus is crushed with a hook against the anterior wall of the oval window niche. The patient is warned not to react to the sudden noise and possible pain resulting from this surgical step.

c: If correctly broken, the stapes arch has a long anterior and a short posterior crus. Bleeding occurring from the mucosa of the promontory has no adverse effects since the prosthesis is already in situ.

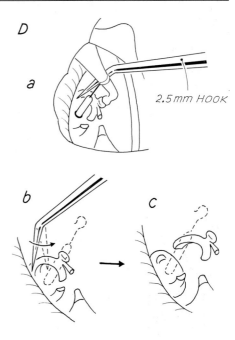

Fig. 114

Checking final mobility of ossicular chain

After removal of the stapes arch, the correct mobility of the ossicular chain is tested with a 1.5-mm, 45° hook. There should be no free movement of the prosthesis loop when the incus is moved.

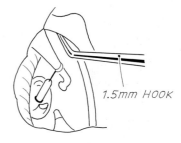

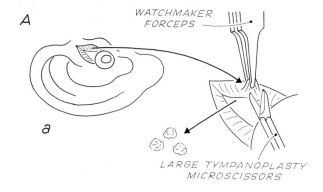

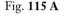

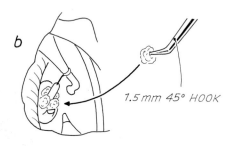

Fig. 115 A

Sealing of stapedotomy opening

a: Connective tissue from the endaural incision is used to seal the stapedotomy opening. Usually, three tissue pledgets are obtained with large tympanoplasty microscissors.

b: Tissue pledgets are placed around the stapedotomy opening using a 1.5-mm, 45° hook and a 0.2-mm footplate elevator.

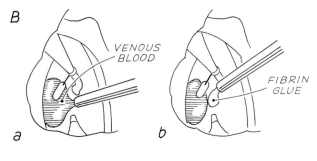

Fig. 115 B

Sealing of stapedotomy opening (cont.)

a: Stapedotomy is very atraumatic so that, usually, there is no accumulation of blood in the oval window at the end of the procedure. Blood is necessary for sealing the fenestrated footplate. Therefore, venous blood is removed at the beginning of the operation from the cubital vein of the patient. The venous blood is stored in a syringe and introduced at this stage of surgery over the connective tissue covering the stapedotomy opening.

b: A drop of fibrin glue is then applied to complete the seal.

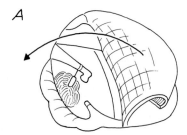

Fig. 116 A

Repositioning the tympanomeatal flap

The tympanomeatal flap is repositioned with a microsuction tube.

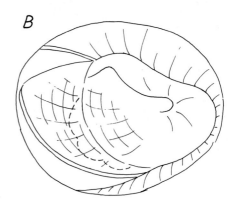

Fig. **116 B**

Repositioning the tympanomeatal flap (cont.)

The bone defect resulting from curetting the canal wall is completely covered by the repositioned tympanomeatal flap. For repair of possible lesions of the tympanomeatal flap see stapedectomy (Figs. 121 A–D, p. 233).

Fig. **117 A**

Packing and wound closure

a: Gelfoam pledgets soaked in Otosporin are used to keep the tympanomeatal flap in place.

b: Note that the Gelfoam is smaller than the diameter of the external canal to avoid excessive pressure on the tympanic membrane after swelling.

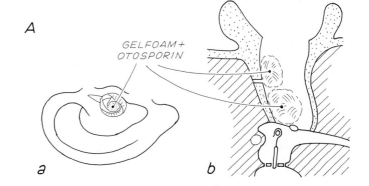

Fig. **117 B**

Packing and wound closure (cont.)

The endaural incision is closed with two 4–0 Ethibond sutures. A strip of gauze impregnated with Terracortril ointment is introduced into the lateral external canal. The packing is left in place for 2 to 4 days.

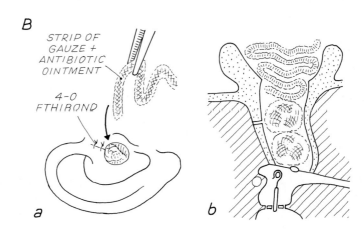

2. Stapedectomy

Surgical Technique

Stapedectomy is used when a limited central perforation of the footplate (stapedotomy) is impossible. This is the case when there is an inadvertent fracture of the footplate, which does not allow use of manual perforators or when, in a fixed stapes situation, a Spandrel prosthesis is employed.

- Preparation of a wire connective-tissue prosthesis
- Partial or total removal of stapes footplate
- Introduction and fixation of wire connective-tissue prosthesis
- Sealing the oval window with connective tissue, venous blood, and fibrin glue

Surgical Highlights

- Local anesthesia
- Endaural skin incision
- Elevation of the tympanomeatal flap with exposure of the oval window

Surgical Steps

The first steps of stapedectomy, from the skin incision to the preparation of the prosthesis, are similar to those of stapedotomy (see Figs. **107**, **108**, **109** and **110**).

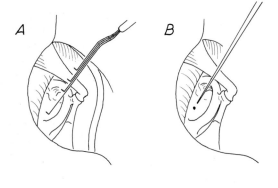

Fig. **118 A**

Determination of prosthesis length

The distance between the footplate and lateral surface of the incus is determined with a malleable measuring rod. The construction of the wire connective-tissue prosthesis is shown in Figs. 119 A–H, p. 230).

Fig. **118 B**

Perforation of the stapes footplate

A small opening is made in the blue central part of the footplate with the 0.3-mm manual perforator (see also Fig. 111 B).

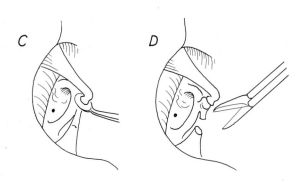

Fig. **118 C**

Separation of the incudostapedial joint

The incudostapedial joint is separated with a joint knife.

Fig. **118 D**

Cutting of the stapedial tendon

The stapedial tendon is cut with small tympanoplasty microscissors.

Fig. 118 E

Removal of stapes arch

The stapes crura are fractured using a 1.5 mm, 90° hook, which is moved away from the fallopian canal. The fractured arch is removed with small alligator forceps.

Fig. 118 F

Hemostasis

Mucosal bleeding may occur after breaking off the stapes arch and is controlled with bipolar microcoagulation (fine angulated microforceps).

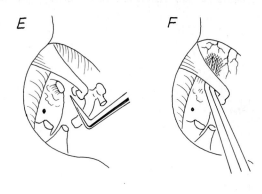

Fig. 118 G

Removal of footplate

The initial opening of the footplate is enlarged superiorly and inferiorly creating two halves of the footplate. The posterior half is removed with a 0.2-mm footplate elevator.

Fig. 118 H

Removal of footplate (cont.)

The anterior half of the footplate is also removed (total stapedectomy).

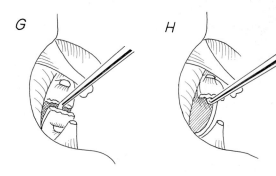

Fig. 118 I

Removal of footplate (cont.)

Surgical site following total removal of the footplate. The macula sacculi is visible in the anterior half of the open oval window.

Fig. 118 J

Introduction of prosthesis

The wire connective-tissue prosthesis is introduced and crimped over the long process of the incus. Large straight alligator forceps are used for this purpose. Small straight alligator forceps are also used for the final adaptation of the wire loop. The top of the loop should conform to the incus properly. A deformed wire loop should be removed and replaced by a new prosthesis.

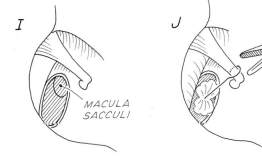

MACULA SACCULI

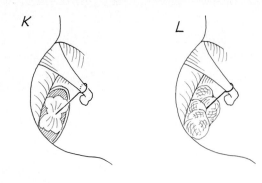

Fig. 118 K

Introduction of prosthesis (cont.)

The wire connective-tissue prosthesis usually moves forward during crimping and must be repositioned in the center of the oval window. Determination of the correct length and position of the prosthesis is only possible if the connective tissue attached to the prosthesis foot is smaller than the lumen of the oval window.

Fig. 118 L

Sealing of oval window

Four small pieces of connective tissue are placed over the open areas of the oval window. Further sealing is obtained with venous blood and fibrin glue (see also Fig. 115 B).

The further steps of stapedectomy (repositioning of the tympanomeatal flap, packing, and wound closure) are performed as for stapedotomy (see Figs. **116** and **117 A–B**).

2.1 Construction of Wire Connective-Tissue Prosthesis

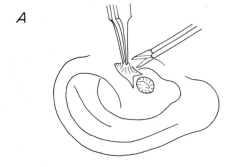

Fig. 119 A

Harvesting of connective tissue

A piece of connective tissue is excised from the original endaural incision using a pair of watch-maker forceps and large tympanoplasty microscissors.

Fig. 119 B

Fixation of connective tissue to the stainless steel wire

The connective tissue is fixed by the scrub nurse with watchmaker forceps. A 0.005-inch stainless steel wire is tied tightly across the middle of the connective tissue.

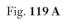

0.005 STAINLESS
STEEL WIRE

Fig. 119 C

Use of wire-bending die

The wire is looped around the larger of two posts of a wire-bending die. By pulling on the wire, the desired length of the prosthesis is established. The left portion of the wire is then rotated inferiorly to the right until a proper loop is formed along the smaller post.

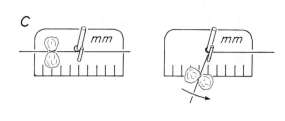

Fig. 119 D

Formation of the prosthesis loop

The wire is removed from the posts of the wire-bending die. The loop of the wire is adapted to the size of the long process of the incus by introduction of a 1.5-mm, 45°-angled hook into the loop. The loop is then moved along the shaft of the hook with watchmaker forceps until the proper diameter is reached.

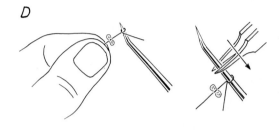

Fig. 119 E

Formation of the prosthesis loop (cont.)

The excess of wire is removed from the loop of the prosthesis with wire cutting scissors.

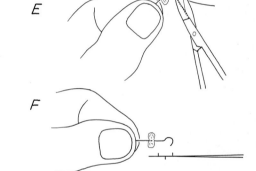

Fig. 119 F

Checking the length of the prosthesis

The length of the prosthesis is checked with a malleable measuring rod.

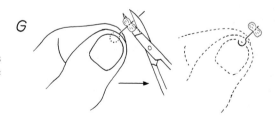

Fig. 119 G

Cutting excess wire

Wire scissors are used to cut the shaft of the wire as close as possible to the knot tied on the connective tissue.

Fig. 119 H

Storage of wire connective-tissue prosthesis

The completed prosthesis is placed on a small gauze impregnated with Ringer's solution and is ready to be grasped with a large straight alligator forceps for introduction into the middle ear.

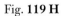
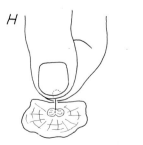

2.2 Alternative Use of a 0.4-mm Teflon Platinum Piston (TPP)

The use of a piston prosthesis in total or partial stapedectomy is dangerous because a lesion of the inner ear membranes may occur if the piston moves to the edge of the oval window while crimping or with delayed migration. Covering the oval window with perichondrium (see Fig. 31 A–C) before placement of the piston avoids these problems, but lateralization of the new oval window membrane may lead to erosion of the incus or migration of the piston. The technique illustrated in the following figures minimizes these risks.

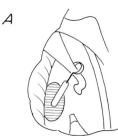

Fig. 120 A

Introduction of the TPP prosthesis

A 0.4-mm TPP is introduced into the center of the open oval window.

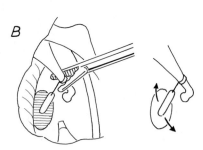

Fig. 120 B

Fixation of prosthesis to incus

The 0.4-mm TPP is crimped to the long process of the incus with large alligator forceps, avoiding as much as possible lateral displacement of the piston.

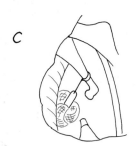

Fig. 120 C

Fixation and sealing of the prosthesis in the center of the oval window

Four pledgets of connective tissue from the endaural incision (see Fig. 115 A) are placed around the piston to keep it centered in the oval window. Sealing is provided by connective tissue, blood from the cubital vein, and fibrin glue.

2.3 Connective-Tissue Graft for Repair of the Tympanomeatal Flap

A perforation or tear may occur during elevation of the tympanomeatal flap in the posterosuperior quadrant of the drum. A gap may also remain between the tympanomeatal flap and the surrounding edge of the incisura Rivini if extensive bone removal has occurred. A connective-tissue graft obtained from the endaural incision is used for repair.

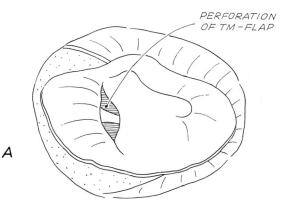

Fig. 121 A

Perforation of tympanomeatal flap

The tympanomeatal flap has been repositioned. The atrophic posterosuperior drum shows a traumatic perforation.

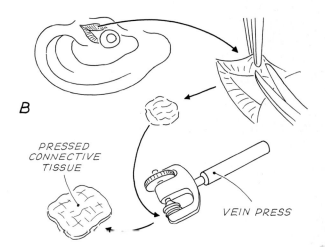

Fig. 121 B

Harvesting and preparation of connective-tissue graft

Connective tissue is obtained from the endaural incision using tissue forceps and curved tympanoplasty scissors. The connective tissue is placed in a Shea vein press. The pressed connective tissue is ready for use.

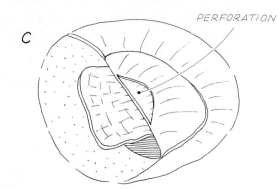

PERFORATION

C

Fig. **121 C**

Underlay of connective-tissue graft

The connective-tissue graft is placed under the drum covering the perforation.

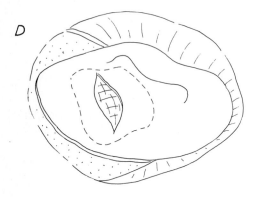

D

Fig. **121 D**

Underlay of connective-tissue graft (cont.)

The broken line shows the position of the underlaid graft.

3. Results (see page 263)

4. Rules and Hints (see page 270)

Chapter 8
Special Applications of Stapes Surgery

1. Incus Replacement with Stapedotomy (IRS) for Malleus and/or Incus Fixation in Otosclerosis

Surgical Technique

Elevating the tympanomeatal flap widely enough to expose the lateral process of the malleus (Fig. **109 C**) permits reliable assessment of mallear mobility at the beginning of stapedotomy or stapedectomy. Revision surgery has shown that failure to initially ex-

pose the short process of the malleus has led the first surgeon to overlook malleus and/or incus fixation in 10% of the cases (see Table **30**). Incus replacement with stapedotomy (IRS) is the method of choice for the functional repair of malleus and/or incus fixation in otosclerosis.

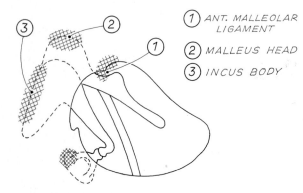

① ANT. MALLEOLAR LIGAMENT

② MALLEUS HEAD

③ INCUS BODY

Fig. **122**

Typical sites of malleus and/or incus fixation in otosclerosis

The most common mallear fixation occurs through ossification of the anterior mallear ligament (**1**). Fixation of the malleus head (**2**) and incus body (**3**) are usually found in narrow external canals.

Surgical Highlights

- Local anesthesia
- Endaural incision
- Elevation of tympanomeatal flap
- Canalplasty
- Removal of incus and malleus head
- Drilling away the ossified anterior mallear ligament
- Introduction of TPP between malleus handle and stapes footplate
- Stapedotomy with manual perforators
- Removal of stapes arch with crurotomy scissors

- Introduction of piston into vestibule
- Fixation of platinum loop to malleus handle
- Sealing of stapedotomy opening

Surgical Steps

The first and last steps of surgery are performed as for stapedotomy (see Figs. **107–110**, pp. 215–220).

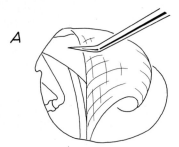

A

Fig. **123 A**

Assessment of mallear mobility

The narrow external canal is widened as shown in Figs. 108 A, B. The tympanomeatal flap is then elevated over the lateral process of the malleus (see Fig. 107 G). Palpation with a 1.5-mm, 45° hook shows that the malleus is completely fixed.

Fig. **123 B**

Separation of incudostapedial joint

A joint knife is used to separate the incudostapedial joint. The mobility of malleus and incus is
assessed again, confirming the mallear fixation.

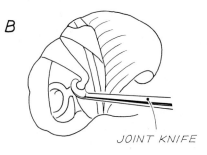

B

JOINT KNIFE

Fig. **123 C**

Exposure of malleus handle

The anterior limb of the tympanomeatal flap is extended to the anterior tympanic spine with tympanoplasty microscissors. The tympanomeatal
flap is elevated from the superior half of the malleus handle using a 2.5-mm, 45° hook. This extended elevation of the tympanomeatal flap avoids
the need to tunnel the space between the malleus
handle and tympanic membrane as proposed in
standard techniques of incus replacement. The
direct view over the malleus handle and stapes footplate facilitates the later introduction of the prosthesis.

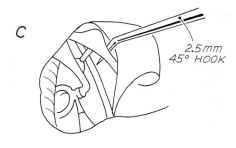

C

*2.5mm
45° HOOK*

Fig. **123 D**

Removal of incus

The incus is mobilized with a 1.5-mm,
45° hook and removed by lateral rotation. Care is taken to preserve the
chorda tympani.

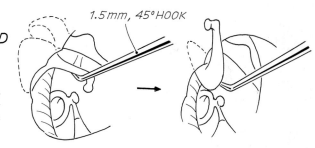

1.5mm, 45°HOOK

D

Fig. **123 E**

Removal of malleus head

A malleus nipper is used to cut the malleus neck. A
0.8-mm diamond burr may be necessary to
achieve transection of the malleus neck when it is
too large.

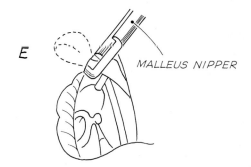

E

MALLEUS NIPPER

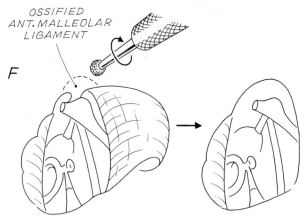

OSSIFIED
ANT. MALLEOLAR
LIGAMENT

F

Fig. **123 F**

Drilling away the ossified anterior mallear ligament

The most common cause of malleus fixation is an ossified anterior mallear ligament. Removal of this ossification is essential for adequate mobilization of the malleus handle and for prevention of its refixation.

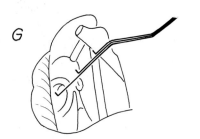

G

Fig. **123 G**

Determination of prosthesis length

A malleable measuring rod is placed between the stapes footplate and the lateral surface of the malleus handle. The tip of the measuring rod may be bent to suit the particular anatomical situation.

Fig. **123 H**

Preparation and introduction of incus replacement prosthesis

The prosthesis for incus replacement is the same as that used for stapedotomy, i. e. the 0.4-mm TPP with a total length (including head) of 7 or 9 mm (see Figs. 110 B–C, page 220). The loop is shaped like that of a clothes hanger to help insertion over the malleus handle and facilitates closing the loop with a hook when direct adaptation with small alligator forceps is impossible. The TPP is trimmed on the cutting block and is introduced with large alligator forceps between the footplate and malleus handle, remaining inferior to the chorda tympani. The length of the prosthesis is correct if the loop exceeds the level of the malleus handle by 0.5 mm. A longer prosthesis has to be trimmed again on the cutting block. A short prosthesis has to be replaced.

H

I

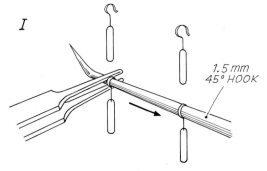

1.5 mm
45° HOOK

Fig. **123 I**

Adaptation of the prosthesis loop to the size of the malleus handle

The malleus neck may be larger than the incus. In this case, the loop of the prosthesis is enlarged by moving it along a 1.5-mm, 45° hook with watchmaker forceps.

Fig. 123 J

Perforation of the footplate

After the correct length of the prosthesis has been assessed, the TPP is
moved out of the oval window. An
opening slightly larger than 0.4 mm
is made in the center of the footplate
as for stapedotomy (see Fig. 111 B)
using manual perforators.

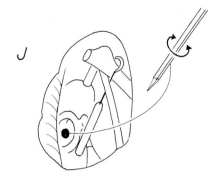

Fig. 123 K

Removal of the stapes arch

The stapes arch is removed
after stapedotomy to avoid
destabilization of the footplate.
Crurotomy scissors are used to
cut the posterior (a) and anterior (b) crus. The posterior crus
must be cut as short as possible
to facilitate introduction of the
Teflon piston (c).

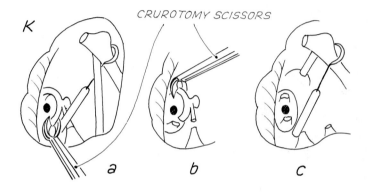

CRUROTOMY SCISSORS

a   b   c

Fig. 123 L

Introduction and fixation of the prosthesis

The TPP is introduced into the vestibule. The prosthesis loop is adapted
to the malleus handle by means of
small straight alligator forceps.

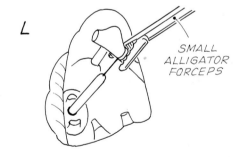

SMALL
ALLIGATOR
FORCEPS

Fig. 123 M

Sealing of stapedotomy opening

The stapedotomy open-
ing (a) is sealed with connective-tissue pledgets (b),
blood, and fibrin glue (c).

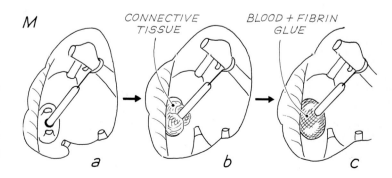

CONNECTIVE
TISSUE

BLOOD + FIBRIN
GLUE

a   b   c

2. Obliterative Otosclerosis

Obliterative otosclerosis is found in 13.7% of primary cases (see page 263).

Surgical Technique

The first and last steps of the procedure are performed as for stapedotomy (see Figs. **107–110**, pp. 215–220) and **116 A–B**, pp. 226–7).

Surgical Highlights

- Local anesthesia
- Endaural incision
- Elevation of tympanomeatal flap
- Exposure of oval window
- Removal of stapes arch
- Removal of obliterative focus with diamond burr
- Exposure of a blue area in the central oval window
- Determination of prosthesis length and trimming
- Formation of a stapedotomy opening
- Introduction and fixation of prosthesis
- Sealing of stapedotomy opening with connective tissue, venous blood, and fibrin glue

Surgical steps

Fig. **124 A**

Surgical site in obliterative otosclerosis

The stapes arch is removed as for stapedectomy. A large promontorial otosclerotic focus obliterates the inferior half of the oval window niche. The remaining stapes footplate is also thickened by otosclerosis. If the space between the facial nerve and stapes arch allows introduction of the 0.6-mm diamond burr, the obliterative focus is drilled away and a stapedotomy opening is created with the stapes arch in place. Otherwise, the stapes arch is removed as in stapedectomy, following separation of the incudostapedial joint using a 1-mm, 90° hook (Fig. 118 E).

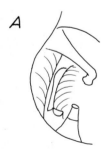

A

Fig. 124 B

Drilling away the obliterative focus

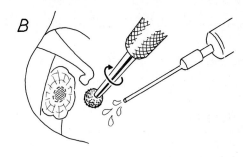

A 0.8-mm diamond burr is used to remove the excess of promontorial bone saucerizing the oval window niche until a blue area of slightly more than 0.4-mm in diameter is exposed in the center of the oval window. The correct size of the blue area is determined with a malleable 0.4-mm caliper rod. Drilling is performed using the Micro-Mega handpiece (N. 117 013), which is thin enough for all types of endaural surgery. Care is taken to avoid irrigation (and therefore contamination) through the external auditory canal. Irrigation is performed by means of a syringe filled with Ringer's solution carrying a microsuction tube, which is directly introduced into the middle ear. Drilling and irrigation are not performed simultaneously, but sequentially, because the left hand carries the microsuction tube while drilling.

Fig. 124 C

Determination of prosthesis length

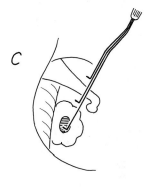

The length of the prosthesis is determined *after* exposure of the blue area in the center of the oval window.

Fig. 124 D

Perforation of the oval window

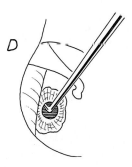

The exposed blue bone is removed with a 0.6-mm diamond burr until the endosteum is exposed. The speed of the burr is reduced for this purpose. Only burrs having a perfect concentric rotation should be used. The slightest distortion of the burr's shaft producing eccentric rotation does not allow precise work. The last layer of shattered bone covering the 0.4-mm opening is removed with a 0.2-mm footplate elevator. The footplate elevator is bent to conform to the anatomical situation.

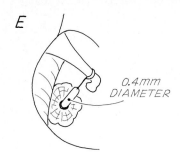

Fig. **124 E**

Introduction and fixation of TPP

The TPP is trimmed on the cutting block (Figs. 110 B, C), introduced with straight alligator forceps into the middle ear, and advanced 0.5 mm into the vestibule. The prosthesis loop is attached to the incus with straight alligator forceps.

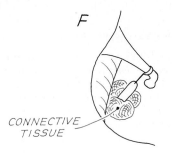

Fig. **124 F**

Sealing of stapedotomy opening

Connective-tissue pledgets, venous blood, and fibrin glue are used to seal the stapedotomy opening. Adequate sealing is important in obliterative otosclerosis because the stapedotomy opening is made larger than in conventional surgery. With a small hole, the thickness of the surrounding bone could prevent free movements of the prosthesis.

3. Floating Footplate

A floating footplate may occur after disruption of the stapes arch when a thick otosclerotic footplate is minimally fixed to the annular ligament. Reversal of the conventional steps of stapes surgery with drilling of the footplate with the intact incudo-stapedial joint and stapes arch has considerably reduced the incidence of a floating footplate. The complication may still occur in biscuit-type otosclerotic footplates, which do not permit central perforation before the stapes arch is broken. This occurs in less than 1% of the cases.

Surgical Technique

The first and last steps of surgery are performed as for stapedotomy (see Figs. **107–110,** pp. 215–220 and **116 A–B,** pp. 226–7).

Surgical Highlights

- Drilling a small opening at the inferior margin of the oval window niche with a 0.6 mm diamond burr
- Extraction of the footplate with hook through the inferior burr hole

Surgical Steps

In the illustrated case, the first steps of the procedures were performed as for stapedotomy. The stapes arch was then removed because there was insufficient space for a 0.6-mm burr between facial nerve and stapes suprastructure.

Fig. 125 A

Attempted extraction with two hooks

One hook (left hand) stabilizes the posterior crus. A second hook (right hand) is slipped under the inferior margin of the footplate, to try to elevate it out of the oval window. Rotation of the footplate within the vestibule is dangerous. Therefore, the inferior hook should be introduced under the central portion of the footplate to lateralize it without medial rotation of the superior margin into the .vestibule.

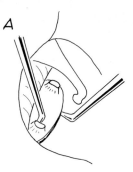

A

Fig. 125 B

Drilling of a burr hole at the inferior edge of the oval window

If extraction with two hooks is impossible, a small burr hole is drilled along the inferior margin of the oval window using a 0.6-mm diamond burr. The burr hole is just large enough to introduce the tip of a 0.5-mm, 45° hook.

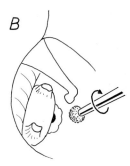

B

Fig. 125 C

Extraction of floating footplate

The footplate is extracted as described in Fig. 125 A. In case of difficult extraction or of inexperience, the surgeon is better advised to back out from the procedure. The operation can then be carried out by a more experienced surgeon after refixation has occurred (6–12 months later).

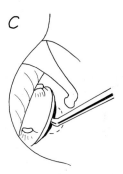

C

4. Narrow Oval Window Niche

Surgical Technique

A narrow oval window niche is often the result of a prominent or dehiscent facial nerve covering the majority of the footplate.

    The first steps of surgery are performed as for stapedotomy (Figs. **107–110**, pp. 215–220). The stapes arch is removed as for stapedectomy (Fig. **118 E**, p. 229).

Surgical Highlights

- Enlargement of the oval window niche with a diamond burr
- Stapedotomy or
- removal of incus and incus replacement with stapedotomy

Surgical Steps

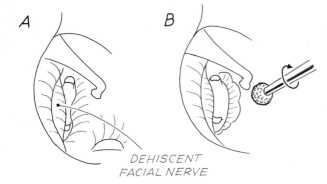

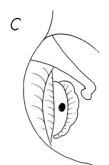

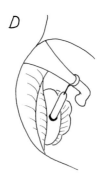

DEHISCENT
FACIAL NERVE

Fig. 126 A

Surgical site following removal of the stapes arch

The facial nerve is dehiscent. The stapes arch obscures the footplate and was removed with crurotomy scissors.

Fig. 126 B

Enlargement of oval window niche

The excess of promontorial bone is removed with a 0.8-mm diamond burr until the inferior half of the footplate is visible.

Fig. 126 C

Stapedotomy

A 0.4-mm opening is made with manual perforators (in a blue footplate) or with a 0.6-mm diamond burr in a white, thickened footplate.

Fig. 126 D

Introduction and fixation of TPP

A 0.4-mm TPP is introduced into the stapedotomy opening. The prosthesis loop is firmly attached to the incus. The stapedotomy hole is sealed with connective tissue, venous blood, and fibrin glue.

Fig. **126 E**

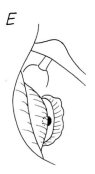

Subtotal obstruction of oval window by dehiscent facial nerve

In the presence of a very prominent and dehiscent facial nerve, the incus is removed because the mobility of the TPP would be hampered. The 0.4-mm opening is partially made under the nerve with manual perforators. This is a situation in which the use of a laser is impractical!

Fig. **126 F**

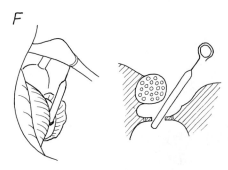

Incus replacement with stapedotomy

The 0.4-mm TPP is attached to the malleus handle and advanced for 0.5 mm in the vestibule. The mobility of the Teflon piston remains free due to the anterior inclination of the prosthesis. The stapedotomy opening is larger than usual to account for the angulation of the piston.

5. Short Incus

A short incus creates the problem of possible contact between the prosthesis and facial nerve.

Surgical Technique

The first and last steps of the procedure are performed as for stapedotomy (see Figs. **107**–**110**, pp. 215–220 and **116 A**–**B**, pp. 226–7).

Surgical Highlights

- Bending of the prosthesis shaft to overcome the bulge of the facial nerve or
- Removal of the incus and incus replacement with stapedotomy

Surgical Steps

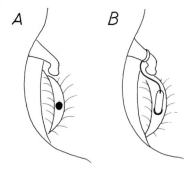

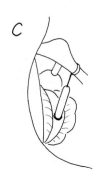

Fig. **127 A**

Surgical site with short incus

The 0.4-mm stapedotomy was performed after the stapes arch was removed.

Fig. **127 B**

Stapedotomy with modified prosthesis

The platinum shaft of the 0.4-mm TPP has been bent in situ between two hooks to overcome the bulge of the dehiscent facial nerve. The modification of the prosthesis is technically more difficult and the results are not as good as those of incus replacement with stapedotomy (see next Figure).

Fig. **127 C**

Incus replacement with stapedotomy

The anteroinferior angulation of the prosthesis avoids contact of the piston with the facial nerve. The functional results of incus replacement with stapedotomy are similar to those of stapedotomy (see p. 269).

6. Anomalous Facial Nerve

The anomalous facial nerve comes as a surprise during surgery performed for conductive deafness because the auricle, external canal, and tympanic membrane are often normal in appearance. A facial nerve lying over the oval window niche may be associated with an anomaly of the long process of the incus and of the stapes arch. The alternatives for functional restoration of hearing in this situation are (1) the displacement of the facial nerve with *vestibulotomy* and (2) the anterior promontorial *cochleostomy*.

6.1 Vestibulotomy

This operation is performed only if the blue area of the vestibule is visible through the bone after minimal superior displacement of the anomalous tympanic facial nerve. Wide displacement of the facial nerve may be too dangerous, and the operation is not performed under these circumstances.

Surgical Technique

The first and last steps of surgery are performed as for stapedotomy (see Figs. **107– 110**, pp. 215–220 and **116 A–B**, pp. 226–7).

Surgical Highlights

- Removal of the malformed incus and stapes arch
- Minimal superior displacement of the anomalous facial nerve
- Identification of the blue area of the vestibule
- Burr hole in the center of the expected oval window
- Incus replacement and stapedotomy

Surgical Steps

Fig. 128 A

Surgical site with anomalous facial nerve covering the oval window

The long process of the incus and stapes arch is malformed. No oval window is visible.

Fig. 128 B

Identification of the blue area of the vestibule

The facial nerve is gently elevated with the universal microraspatory for a fraction of a millimeter, exposing the bluish area of the vestibule.

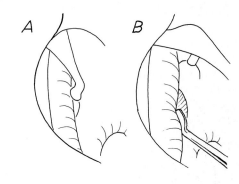

Fig. 128 C

Vestibulotomy

A 0.8-mm diamond burr is used to remove the bone covering the inferior edge of the blue vestibular area. A 0.4-mm opening is performed with a 0.6-mm diamond burr (Bien-Air drill with Micro-Mega handpiece (No. 48 E ORL) in the exposed blue area, close to the facial nerve.

Fig. 128 D

Incus replacement with stapedotomy

A 0.4-mm TPP is attached to the malleus handle and introduced 0.5-mm into the vestibule. Sealing of the oval window, repositioning of the tympanomeatal flap, packing, and wound closure are performed as for stapedotomy.

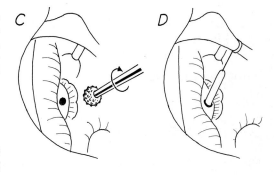

Fig. 128 E

Incorrect placement of prosthesis

Revision surgery showed that an anomalous facial nerve may be interpreted by an inexperienced surgeon as a "polyp" covering the oval window! A Shea Teflon piston introduced through the "polyp" in the vestibule caused immediate facial palsy and total loss of hearing! The piston was removed at revision surgery and the facial nerve widely decompressed to permit recovery of facial function.

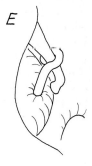

6.2 Promontorial Cochleostomy

A promontorial cochleostomy is performed if exposure of the expected vestibule requires wide displacement of the anomalous facial nerve. The surgical steps for promontorial cochleostomy are shown in the following section.

7. The Missing Stapes

Congenital absence of the stapes is characterized by a total conductive hearing loss. Two anatomical situations are possible: (1) the facial nerve is in the normal position and the oval window identifiable; or (2) the abnormal stapes is associated with an anomalous facial nerve, and the oval window niche is not identifiable. High-resolution CT scans are required to exclude an accompanying inner ear malformation that may lead to a possible gusher or make functional surgery impossible.

Surgical Highlights

- Minimal perforation in the center of the oval window niche to exclude a gusher
- If no gusher: stapedotomy
- In the presence of a gusher: (a) lumbar drainage and stapedotomy or (b) if the patient refuses to accept the risk of total deafness (which is higher than in stapedotomy) the hole made in the footplate is closed and a hearing aid is advised.

7.1 Identifiable Oval Window Niche

Surgical Technique

The operation is carried out with local anesthesia in adults and general anesthesia in children. The first and last steps of the procedure are performed as for stapedotomy (see Figs. **107–110**, pp. 215–220 and **116 A–B,** pp. 226–7).

Surgical Steps

Fig. 129 A

Anomalous stapes with identifiable oval window

The facial nerve in its normal position. The malformed incus was removed. The stapes footplate is missing; the oval window niche is well defined by a depression and bluish discoloration of bone.

Fig. 129 B

Perforation of bone in the center of the oval window niche

A small opening is made in the center of the oval window niche with manual perforators or with a 0.6-mm diamond burr. If a gusher is excluded, stapedotomy is performed.

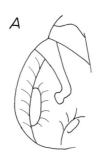
A

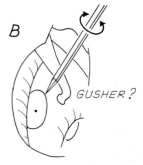
B

GUSHER ?

Fig. 129 C

Stapedotomy

The opening in the center of the oval window is enlarged to a diameter of slightly more than 0.4 mm.

Fig. 129 D

Stapedotomy (cont.)

A 0.4-mm TPP is introduced for 0.5 mm into the vestibule and attached to the incus. The further surgical steps are the same as for stapedotomy (see p. 226).

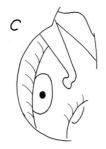
C

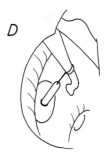
D

Fig. 129 E

Gusher

An extensive outflow of perilymph occurs through the small perforation made in the center of the oval window niche. If the patient has accepted the risks involved with stapedotomy, lumbar drainage is applied.

Fig. 129 F

Gusher (cont.)

The lumbar drainage has stopped the perilymph flow through the stapedotomy opening. The stapedotomy opening is enlarged with manual perforators, and a 0.4-mm TPP is introduced for 0.5 mm into the vestibule and attached to the incus.

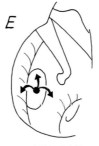
E
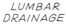

LUMBAR
DRAINAGE

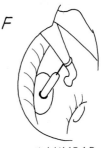
F

+ LUMBAR
DRAINAGE

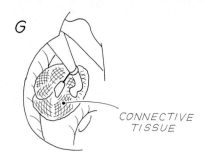

G

CONNECTIVE
TISSUE

Fig. 129 G

Gusher (cont.)

Three pieces of connective tissue from the endaural incision are wrapped around the stapedotomy opening. The connective tissue pieces are large enough to be kept in place by the long process of the incus. Cubital venous blood and fibrin glue are used to supplement the sealing. The intralumbar drain is maintained for 4–5 days.

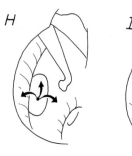

H

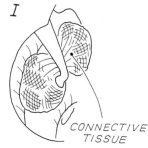

I

CONNECTIVE
TISSUE

Fig. **129 H**

Gusher (cont.)

The patient does not agree to accept the risks involved with a stapedotomy procedure. The operation will be discontinued.

Fig. **129 I**

Gusher (cont.)

The operation is discontinued because the patient has not agreed to accept the risks involved with stapedotomy. The small perforation in the center of the oval window niche is closed with a piece of connective tissue large enough to be firmly secured between the oval window and the incus. Cubital venous blood and fibrin glue supplement the sealing. The patient will be provided with a hearing aid.

7.2 Unidentifiable Oval Window Niche

Surgical Technique

Two alternative techniques are presented:

a) indirectly guided cochleostomy and
b) directly guided cochleostomy

The risk of total deafness in cochleostomy is significantly higher than in stapedotomy. The operation should be carried out by very experienced surgeons. Mobilization of the anomalous facial nerve with vestibulotomy is a further possibility to be discussed with the patient if the anatomic conditions are unfavorable for cochleostomy.

---

* Plester, D., Hildmann, H., Steinbach E. In: Atlas der Ohrchirurgie. Stuttgart: Kohlhammer, 1989.

a) Indirectly Guided Cochleostomy

If the oval window is unidentifiable, fenestration of the scala vestibuli in the basal turn of the cochlea has been advised by Plester*. The landmarks for the 1-mm diameter cochleostomy are given as 1 mm anterior and 1.5 mm inferior to the anterior border of the oval window. These landmarks are difficult to define when the oval window is missing. For this reason we have modified Plester's measurements using the *cochleariform process* as a reference.

Surgical Highlights

- Identification of the cochleariform process
- Cochleostomy performed in the scala vestibuli of the basal turn 1.5 mm below the posterior edge of the cochleariform process
- Incus replacement with stapedotomy

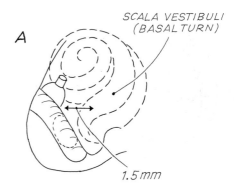

SCALA VESTIBULI (BASAL TURN)

A

1.5 mm

Fig. 130 A

Landmarks for indirect cochleostomy

The upper portion of the scala vestibuli of the basal turn is found 1.5 mm below the posterior edge of the cochleariform process.

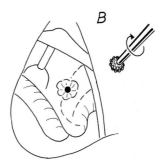

B

Fig. 130 B

Cochleostomy in scala vestibuli of basal turn

The malformed incus and stapes arch were removed. A 0.8-mm diamond burr with suction-irrigation is used to drill the cochleostomy in the scala vestibuli of the basal turn.

Fig. 130 C

Incus replacement with stapedotomy

A 0.4-mm TPP has been trimmed to the proper length, attached to the malleus handle, and introduced into the scala tympani of the basal turn. The piston protrudes 0.2 mm. If there are doubts about the perfect localization of the cochleostomy, the endosteum is not opened and the piston just placed over it.

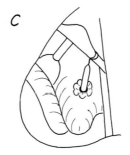

C

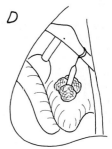

D

b) Directly Guided Cochleostomy

Drilling a cochleostomy on the basis of coordinates only carries a significant risk of sensorineural deafness. For this reason, Dr. J. Buckley** has performed a temporal bone study in our laboratory to determine a more reliable method for cochleostomy. The tech-

nique has been used in a limited number of patients and awaits further confirmation of results.

To date, however, no hearing losses have been observed after directly guided cochleostomy of the scala tympani or vestibuli of the middle turn.

_____

** Janet Nash Clinical Fellow, 1993

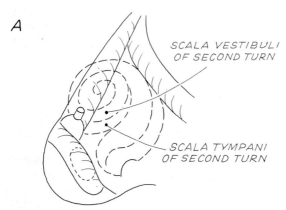

A

SCALA VESTIBULI OF SECOND TURN

SCALA TYMPANI OF SECOND TURN

Fig. **131 A**

Schematic view of cochlear turns

The second turn of the cochlea begins below the anterior part of the cochleariform process and forms an angle of approximately 45° to the semicanal of the tensor tympani muscle.

Fig. **131 B**

Window for cochleostomy in scala vestibuli of middle turn

Drilling of the window is started below the cochleariform process and continued along the lower border of the semicanal of the tensor muscle. The cochlear endosteum is identified at the depth of approximately 1.5 mm. The window has a characteristic appearance, the middle turn being separated from the apical turn by a diagonal bony lamina ("white line") crossing the fenestra obliquely at an angle of 45° to the tensor tympani. The apical turn is superficial to the second turn and is, therefore, encountered first in the anterior part of the bony trough. The bone is removed with a 0.6 mm drill over an area just large enough for a 0.4-mm TPP, remaining as close as possible to the "white line". The distance between the malleus handle and cochleostomy is measured and the TPP cut to size and introduced as for incus replacement and stapedotomy. The direction of the piston is angled slightly away from the cochlear duct, further reducing the risks of injury. In view of the minimal distance of 0.48 mm, the use of a 0.4-mm diameter piston is essential. If in doubt about the position of the cochleostomy, the endosteum is left intact and the piston placed over it.

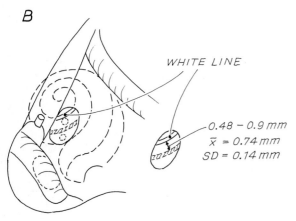

B

WHITE LINE

0.48 – 0.9 mm
$\bar{x}$ = 0.74 mm
SD = 0.14 mm

8. Revision Stapedectomy or Stapedotomy

This section is concerned with the failure to restore conductive hearing with stapedectomy or stapedotomy for otosclerosis.

8.1 Reobliteration of Oval Window

Reobliteration is the most common cause of revision stapedectomy (52% of the cases, see Table **30**). The bone occluding the oval window is usually accompanied by lateral displacement of the prosthesis. The surgical technique used at revision surgery for the reobliterated oval window is the same as that described for obliterative otosclerosis (see Figs. **124 A–D**, pp. 240–241).

8.2 Migration of Prosthesis Shaft

Displacement of the prosthesis is the second-most frequent complication of stapedectomy.

Surgical Technique

The operation is performed with local anesthesia. The first and last steps of surgery are the same as for stapedotomy (see Figs. **107–110**, pp. 215–220 and **116 A–B**, pp. 226–7).

Surgical Highlights

- Removal of displaced prosthesis
- Exclusion of inner ear lesion
- Central perforation of the membrane covering the oval window
- If no inner ear lesion: stapedotomy
- In the presence of inner ear lesion: no further surgery

Surgical Steps

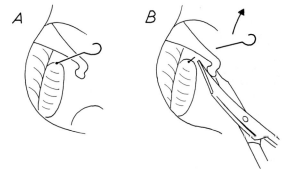

Fig. **132 A**

Migrated wire connective-tissue prosthesis

Stapedectomy with a wire connective-tissue prosthesis was performed 8 years previously. After an initial hearing improvement, the patient experienced a progressive conductive hearing loss over 2 years. The shaft of the prosthesis has migrated anteriorly, and the loop has detached from the incus.

Fig. **132 B**

Removal of prosthesis

The wire is cut close to the oval window membrane with curved tympanoplasty scissors. The wire knot is left in place to avoid the risk of deafness due to intravestibular scars.

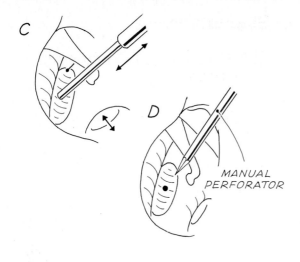

Fig. 132 C

Transmission of perilymphatic movements between oval and round window

A 0.4-mm caliper rod is used to demonstrate the transmission of perilymphatic movements between both windows. Since there is no subjective vertigo when testing the round window reflex, we proceed to stapedotomy.

Fig. 132 D

Perforation of oval window membrane

Manual perforators are used to open the central portion of the oval window membrane.

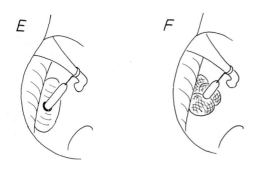

Fig. 132 E

Introduction of prosthesis

A 0.4-mm TPP is introduced for 0.5 mm into the vestibule and its loop attached to the incus.

Fig. 132 F

Sealing of stapedotomy opening

Connective-tissue pledgets, cubital venous blood, and fibrin glue are used to seal the opening in the oval window membrane. Scarifying the mucous membrane of the oval window niche facilitates taking of the connective-tissue grafts.

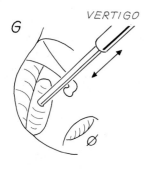

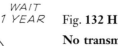

Fig. 132 G

Presence of vertigo or absent round window reflex

The 0.4-mm caliper rod does not induce transmission of perilymphatic movements between both windows. The patient complains about vertigo when the oval window membrane is palpated.

Fig. 132 H

No transmission of perilymphatic movements between both windows

In the presence of vertigo and in the absence of movements between both windows, no further surgery is performed. The patient will be supplied with a hearing aid.

8.3 Detachement of Prosthesis Loop

This situation is frequently due to the insufficient adaptation of the prosthesis loop to the incus.

Surgical Steps

Fig. **133**

Refixation of prosthesis loop

A stapedotomy with a TPP was performed 1 year previously. The operation left a conductive hearing loss of 30 dB.

a: Revision surgery reveals an insufficient adaptation of the prosthesis loop to the incus.

b: Prosthesis length being correct, the Teflon piston is pushed into the stapedotomy opening and the prosthesis loop correctly reattached to the incus with straight alligator forceps.

Surgical Technique

The first and last steps of surgery are carried out as for stapedotomy (see Figs. **107–110**, pp. 215–220 and **116 A–B**, pp. 226–7).

Surgical Highlights

- Refixation of prosthesis loop

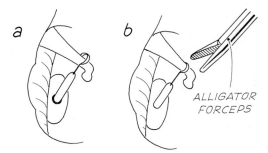

a   b

ALLIGATOR FORCEPS

8.4 Overly Long Prosthesis

According to the condition of the incus, different ossicular situations may be distinguished.

a) Incus Intact

Surgical Technique

The operation is performed with local anesthesia. The first and last surgical steps are the same as for stapedotomy (see Figs. **107–110**, pp. 215–220 and **116 A–B**, pp. 226–7).

Surgical Highlights

- Old prosthesis is replaced by a new one

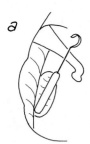
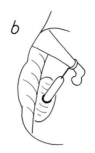

Surgical Steps

Fig. **134**

Replacement of old prosthesis

A wire Teflon piston that is too long had been introduced 2 years previously. After total stapedectomy, the oval window was covered with compressed perichondrium. Some hearing improvement was achieved, but the conductive hearing loss recurred. The 0.6-mm wire Teflon piston had migrated posteriorly. The loop was detached from the incus and ready to extrude through the tympanic membrane. The old prosthesis was removed and a 0.4-mm TPP is now introduced into the vestibule.

b) Erosion of Incus

This type of complication is most commonly found after a polyethylene strut or old Teflon piston has been used.

Surgical Technique

The operation is performed with local anesthesia. The first and last steps are the same as in stapedotomy (see Figs. **107–110**, pp. 215–220 and **116 A–B**, pp. 226–7).

Surgical Highlights

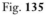

- Incus replacement with stapedotomy

Surgical Steps

Fig. **135**

Incus replacement with stapedotomy

The old Teflon piston introduced 3 years previously has led to complete erosion of the long process of the incus. This lesion is probably due to pressure exerted by the memory of the prosthesis loop. The prosthesis and the incus were removed. An opening is made in the center of the oval window membrane with manual perforators (see Fig. 132 D). A 0.4-mm TPP is attached to the malleus handle and introduced 0.5 mm into the vestibule.

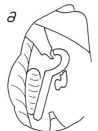
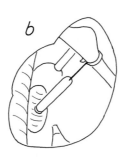

8.5 Previously Undetected Malleus and/or Incus Fixation

This situation is encountered even in repeated revision surgery. This emphasizes the need for complete exposure of the lateral process of the malleus at initial surgery. The repair technique is similar to that of incus replacement with stapedotomy (see Figs. **123 A–M**).

8.6 Perilymph Fistula

A perilymph fistula may occur following any type of stapes surgery. There is no reliable test to detect a perilymph fistula. Fluctuation of hearing and vertigo are the most common clinical symptoms associated with a perilymph fistula.

Surgical Technique

The first and last steps of surgery are similar to those of stapedotomy (see Figs. **107–110**, pp. 215–220 and **116 A–B**, pp. 226–7).

Surgical Highlights

- Removal of previous prosthesis
- Inner ear function preserved: closure of the perilymph fistula with reconstruction of the ossicular chain
- No inner ear function: closure of fistula without reconstruction of ossicular chain, reevaluation after a year

Surgical Steps

Fig. **136 A**

Perilymph fistula following stapedectomy

a: Surgical site 8 years following stapedectomy with a 0.6-mm wire Teflon piston. A fluctuating sensorineural hearing loss and vertigo appeared following an alpine car ride.

b: A similar situation 5 years following a stapedectomy with a connective-tissue wire prosthesis. A sudden hearing loss occurred immediately following an airplane flight. The probable cause of the fistula was excessive movement of the incus with elevation of the piston out of the vestibule.

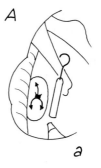
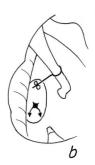

A

a

b

Fig. **136 B**

Removal of prosthesis

The wire loop is detached from the incus with a 1.5-mm, 45° hook. The wire knot was easily separated from the fat tissue covering the oval window, and the prosthesis was removed.

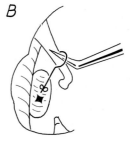

B

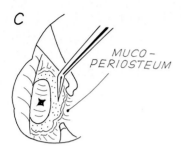

Fig. **136 C**

Creation of a raw surface at the oval window niche

The mucosa surrounding the oval window is scraped away to create a raw surface, which facilitates the taking of perichondrium used for closure of the fistula.

Fig. **136 D**

Closure of perilymph fistula with tragal perichondrium

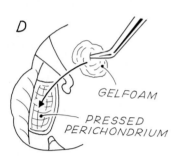

Pressed tragal perichondrium (see Fig. 31 B, p. 65) is placed over the oval window and the surrounding raw surface of mucosa. Gelfoam pledgets soaked in Ringer's solution are placed between the perichondrium and the incus to keep the former in place. Venous blood from the patient and fibrin glue provide further fixation of the seal. A stapedotomy with a 0.4-mm TPP may be performed a year later if inner ear function has recovered.

9. Stapedotomy in Fenestrated Ears

Fenestrated ears are found in patients operated on for otosclerosis before 1958. The condition is therefore becoming increasingly rare. Revision surgery is indicated in the presence of an air–bone gap of more than 30 dB.

Surgical Technique

The operation is performed with local anesthesia. The first and last steps are similar to those of stapedotomy (Figs. **107–110,** pp. 215–220 and **116 A–B,** pp. 226–7).

Surgical Highlights

- Incus replacement with stapedotomy
- Closure of fenestra with bone dust, fibrin glue, and conchal cartilage

Surgical Steps

Fig. **137 A**

Revision surgery following fenestration

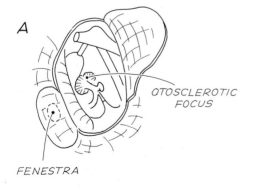

The tympanomeatal flap is raised. The incus and malleus head were removed previously. The stapes is fixed by a large anterior otosclerotic focus. The fenestra of the lateral semicircular canal is visible under the covering skin.

Fig. 137 B

Incus replacement with stapedotomy

The stapes arch and the anterior otosclerotic focus were removed with crurotomy scissors and a 0.6-mm burr (Micro-Mega handpiece No. 48 E ORL). The incus replacement with stapedotomy was performed using a 0.4-mm TPP.

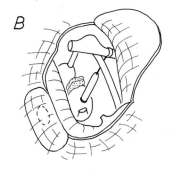

B

Fig. 137 C

Exposure of fenestra of the lateral semicircular canal

The stapedotomy opening is sealed with connective tissue, venous blood, and fibrin glue. A skin flap is raised over the lateral semicircular canal, exposing the fenestra. Care is taken to leave the membrane covering the lumen of the fenestra intact.

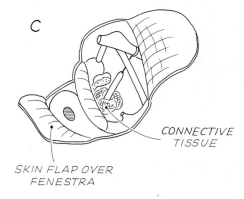

C

CONNECTIVE TISSUE

SKIN FLAP OVER FENESTRA

Fig. 137 D

Two-layer closure of fenestra

Bone dust impregnated with fibrin glue (bone paste) covers the fenestra nov-ovalis.

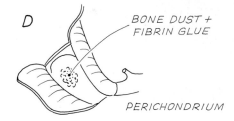

D

BONE DUST + FIBRIN GLUE

PERICHONDRIUM

Fig. 137 E

Two-layer closure of fenestra (cont.)

A piece of conchal cartilage with attached perichondrium is obtained from the posterior surface of the pinna (see Fig. 54). The cartilage is cut to the desired size. The perichondrium is used to stabilize the conchal cartilage over the fenestra.

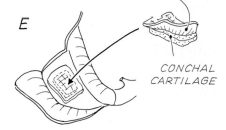

E

CONCHAL CARTILAGE

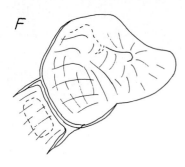

F

Fig. **137 F**

Repositioning of the tympanomeatal flap

The skin flap over the lateral canal and the tympanomeatal flap are repositioned. Gelfoam pledgets soaked in Otosporin are used to keep both flaps in place.

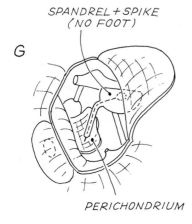

SPANDREL + SPIKE
(NO FOOT)

G

PERICHONDRIUM

Fig. **137 G**

Alternative procedure: total stapedectomy with Spandrel II

A total stapedectomy is performed and the oval window covered with pressed tragal perichondrium. A Spandrel II with spike but no shoe (see Fig. 31 D–I) is introduced between the oval window and the undersurface of the drum just posterior to the malleus handle.

In our experience, both techniques, the incus replacement with stapedotomy and the total stapedectomy with Spandrel, have achieved an average air–bone gap closure to 20–30 dB. This is probably due to the difficulty in achieving bony closure of the lateral canal fenestra. The results of incus replacement with stapedotomy are more reliable in the long term.

10. Stapes Surgery in Tympanosclerosis

Total or partial removal of the footplate in tympanosclerosis is considered to have a high risk of postoperative total hearing loss. In our experience, this is not the case if the operation is staged.

Surgical Technique

The first stage (closed mastoido-epitympanectomy with tympanoplasty) is carried out under general anesthesia. The second stage follows 6–12 months later with local anesthesia. The surgical steps are similar to those for stapedotomy (see Figs. **107–110**, pp. 215–220).

Surgical Highlights

- Second stage
- Local anesthesia
- Incus replacement with stapedotomy or
- Stapedectomy with Spandrel II

Surgical Steps

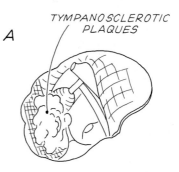

A

TYMPANOSCLEROTIC PLAQUES

Fig. 138 A

Surgical site at second stage

The incus and malleus were removed at first surgery. The stapes is surrounded by massive tympanosclerotic plaques.

Fig. 138 B

Removal of tympanosclerosis from the oval window niche

The stapes arch is removed with a 0.6-mm diamond burr (Micro-Mega handpiece, No. 1170/3). The tympanosclerotic plaques within the oval window niche are gently elevated with a 0.5-mm, 45° hook, exposing a fixed but blue footplate. This is a very common finding in tympanosclerosis. After exposure of the bluish central footplate, the removal of tympanosclerotic plaques is stopped to avoid mobilization of the footplate.

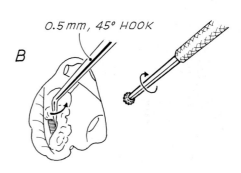

0.5 mm, 45° HOOK

B

Fig. 138 C

Exposed footplate

View over the exposed blue footplate.

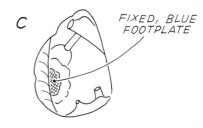

C

FIXED, BLUE FOOTPLATE

Fig. 138 D

Perforation of footplate

Manual perforators are used to form a 0.4-mm opening in the fixed footplate.

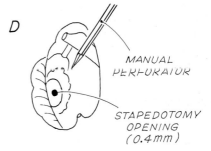

D

MANUAL PERFORATOR

STAPEDOTOMY OPENING (0.4 mm)

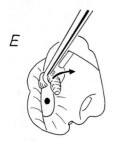

E

Fig. **138 E**

Removal of residual tympanosclerotic plaques from the oval window

After perforation of the footplate, the remaining tympanosclerotic plaques are removed from the edge of the oval window with a 0.2-mm footplate elevator. In this way, restriction of the movements of the TPP is avoided. The possible mobilization of the footplate does not matter at this stage because the stapedotomy opening has already been made.

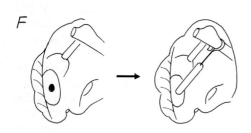

F

Fig. **138 F**

Incus replacement with stapedotomy

A 0.4-mm TPP is introduced into the vestibule and attached to the malleus.

Alternative Procedure: Stapedectomy with Spandrel II

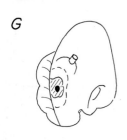

G

Fig. **138 G**

Surgical site following perforation of the footplate

A hole is made in the central footplate with a manual perforator.

0.2 mm FOOTPLATE ELEVATOR

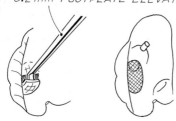

H

Fig. **138 H**

Total stapedectomy

The footplate is extracted in various pieces using a 0.2-mm footplate elevator.

SPANDREL + SPIKE
(NO FOOT)

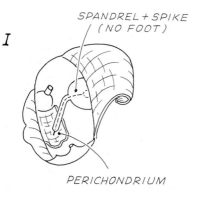

I

Fig. **138 I**

Introduction of the Spandrel II

The opened oval window is covered with pressed tragal perichondrium. A Spandrel II with spike but no shoe is introduced between the perichondrium and the drum (see also Fig. 31 D–G, p. 66).

PERICHONDRIUM

11. Results of Stapes Surgery

11.1 Stapedectomy versus 0.6-mm Stapedotomy

340 patients submitted to primary surgery were divided in two groups of 170 patients each (Table **19**).
The technique of *stapedectomy* with a wire connective-tissue prosthesis was used in one group, and the technique of *stapedotomy* with a 0.6-mm wire Teflon piston was used in the other group of patients.
Both groups of patients presented with a homogeneous distribution of age, sex, and preoperative hearing.
The distribution of oval window pathology was: rim, 78.8%; biscuit, 7.5%; obliterative, 13.7%.

The postoperative success of the operation was measured by analyzing the average postoperative air–bone gap for the speech frequencies (500 Hz, 1000 Hz and 2000 Hz). For 4000 Hz, the postoperative air conduction was compared to the preoperative bone conduction.
The significance of differences in the results were analyzed by the biostatistical center of the University of Zurich, using the Wilcoxon test.
Tables **20**–**24** show that there is no statistical difference between stapedectomy and stapedotomy with regard to the results obtained for the average speech frequencies. There is a constant improvement in the results during the first 3 postoperative months. Thereafter,

Table **19**   Preoperative air conduction versus type of prosthesis

Preoperative bone conduction (dB)	Connective-tissue wire prosthesis (CTW) n = 170			Wire teflon piston (WTP) n = 170		
	n	%	Mean preoperative air conduction (dB)	n	%	Mean preoperative air conduction (dB)
0–20	86	50.6	55.1	92	54.1	56.5
21–40	74	43.5	68.5	67	39.4	71.7
41–60	10	5.9	90.5	11	6.5	87.4

Table **20**   0–5 dB postoperative air–bone gap versus type of prosthesis

Postoperative follow up	CTW n	%	WTP n	%	p	Total number of cases
3 weeks	14/62	22.6	9/61	14.7	NS	123
3 months	38/100	38.0	28/102	27.5	NS	202
1 year	27/86	31.4	23/103	22.3	p < 0.1	189
3 years	8/33	24.2	11/33	33.3	NS	66
4 years or more	14/43	32.5	0/2	0	NS	45

Table **21** 0–10 dB postoperative air–bone gap versus type of prosthesis

Postoperative follow-up	CTW n	%	WTP n	%	p	Total number of cases
3 weeks	27/62	43.5	23/61	37.7	NS	123
3 months	58/100	58.0	52/102	51.0	NS	202
1 year	46/86	53.5	60/103	58.3	NS	189
3 years	19/33	57.6	17/33	51.5	NS	66
4 years or more	26/43	60.5	0/2	0	p < 0.1	45

Table **22** 0–20 dB postoperative air–bone gap versus type of prosthesis

Postoperative follow-up	CTW n	%	WTP n	%	p	Total number of cases
3 weeks	53/62	85.5	43/61	70.5	p < 0.05	123
3 months	83/100	83.0	83/102	81.4	NS	202
1 year	72/86	83.7	85/103	82.5	NS	189
3 years	28/33	84.8	28/33	84.8	NS	66
4 years or more	38/43	88.3	2/2	100	NS	45

Table **23** 30 dB postoperative air–bone gap versus type of prosthesis

Postoperative follow-up	CTW n	%	WTP n	%	p	Total number of cases
3 weeks	2/62	3.2	6/61	9.8	NS	123
3 months	6/100	6.0	6/102	5.9	NS	202
1 year	3/86	3.5	5/103	4.9	NS	189
3 years	3/33	9.0	4/33	12.1	NS	66
4 years or more	1/43	2.3	0/2	0	NS	45

Table **24** Air–bone gap at 4000 Hz 1 year post-operative

Air–bone gap (dB)	CTW n	%	WTP n	%	p
0–5	18/72	25.0	31/74	41.8	< 0.05
0–10	32/73	43.8	45/74	60.8	< 0.05

no change in hearing is observed for as long as 4 years. This confirms previous observations made by Fisch and Rüedi.

The results obtained with both surgical techniques in rim fixation are comparable. Stapedotomy gives the expected superior results in obliterative otosclerosis.

The best success is found in patients under 50 years of age with rim fixation and preoperative bone conduction of 20 to 40 dB. The worst results are seen in patients over 50 years of age with biscuit or obliterative oval window pathology and a preoperative bone conduction of 40–60 dB.

11.2 Stapedotomy (0.4 mm)

The 0.4-mm TPP has been used systematically since 1978. The experience gained with the 0.4-mm TPP has led to the development of a 0.4-mm wire and later to the Platinum Band Teflon Piston. With the slimmer shaft prosthesis, it was possible to reverse the conventional steps of surgery and to fenestrate the footplate, leaving the stapes arch in place (see p. 221). The comparison of the results for 0.5 kHz to 2 kHz obtained in 52 patients operated upon with a 0.6-mm and 0.4-mm stapedotomy, who were followed up for at least 1 year are shown in Tables 25 and 26.

The 0.4-mm stapedotomy yielded poorer results 3 weeks postoperatively, but there was no significant difference in the results of both the 0.6-mm and 0.4-mm techniques, at 3 months and 1 year follow-up. This indicates that a 0.4-mm diameter stapedotomy needs more time to be ultimately successful than a larger diameter stapedotomy. The delay needed to achieve the final hearing level must be considered to avoid untimely disappointment when comparing results of prostheses with various diameters. A 0.3-mm piston needs a delay of 2 to 3 years to reach the final hearing result (G. D. L. Smith, TH Hassard)[*]; 0.4 mm is, therefore, the minimal diameter that can be used for successful stapes surgery. No statistical difference was found for the 0.6-mm and 0.8-mm piston at 4 kHz (Table 27).

Figures 139 and 140 show the 5-year postoperative results of 235 0.4-mm

---

[*] Smith GDL, Hassard TH. Eighteen Years of Experience with Stapedotomy, the Case of the Small Fenestra Operation. Ann Otol Rhinol Laryngol 1978 (Suppl. 49): 87.

Table 25 0–5 dB postoperative air–bone gap (0.5–2 kHz)[*]

Follow-up time	Stapedotomy (0.6 mm, %)	Stapedotomy (0.4 mm, %)	p
3 weeks	15	0	<0.05
3 months	28	14	NS
1 year	22	28	NS

[*] Averaged 0–5 dB postoperative air–bone gap (0.5–2 kHz, n = 52). Note that the results for the 0.4-mm Wire Teflon Piston are poorer 3 weeks postoperatively. However, there is no difference between the hearing obtained 3 months and 1 year following surgery with the 0.4-mm and the 0.6-mm stapedotomy. Fisch, U. Am J Otol. 1982;4(2):112–117.

Table 26 0–10 dB postoperative air–bone gap (0.5–2 kHz)[*]

Follow-up time	Stapedotomy (0.6 mm, %)	Stapedotomy (0.4 mm, %)	p
3 weeks	38	16	<0.025
3 months	51	52	NS
1 year	58	45	NS

[*] Averaged 0–10 dB postoperative air–bone gap (0.5–2 kHz, n = 52). Note that the 0.4-mm stapedotomy yields poorer results after 3 weeks. However, there is no statistic difference between the 0.6-mm and 0.4-mm stapedotomy results at the 3 months and 1-year follow-up. Fisch, U. Am J Otol 1982;4(2):112–117.

Table 27 Air–bone gap at 4 kHz (1 year postoperatively)[*]

dB	Stapedotomy (0.6 mm, %)	Stapedotomy (0.4 mm, %)	p
Overclosure	28	36	NS
0–5	49	45	NS
0–10	61	61	NS
Stapedectomy overclosure = 12%			

[*] Note that there is no statistic difference between the results of 0.6-mm and 0.4-mm stapedotomy. The difference between stapedotomy and stapedectomy is particularly evident when the rate of overclosures is compared. Fisch, U. Am J Otol 1982;4(2):112–117.

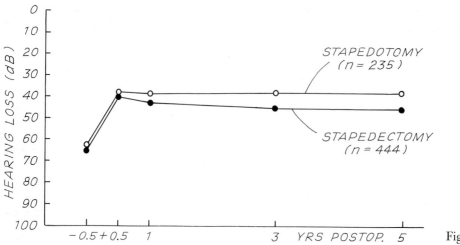

STAPEDECTOMY VS STAPEDOTOMY: AIR CONDUCTION
LEVEL (MEAN OF 0.5, 1, 2 AND 4 KHz)

Fig. **139**

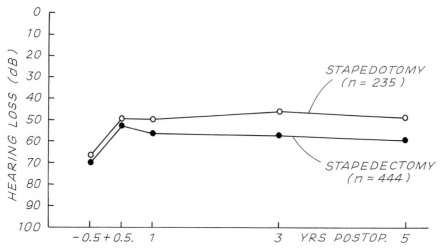

STAPEDECTOMY VS STAPEDOTOMY: AIR CONDUCTION
(4 KHz)

Fig. **140**

stapedotomies and 444 consecutive stapedectomies. The average conductive hearing level for the speech frequencies 0.5–4 kHz diminishes 5.4 dB within five years after stapedectomy and only 0.4 dB after stapedotomy. The average conductive hearing for 4 kHz remains the same for five years after stapedotomy whereas that of stapedectomy is already less in the immediate postoperative period and diminishes by 6.4 dB at the end of 5 years. Therefore, one can say that the long-term results of 0.4-mm stapedotomy are better and more stable than those of stapedectomy, particularly in the upper frequency range.

11.3 Sensorineural Deafness Following Stapes Surgery

A total postoperative deafness occurred in 3 patients after stapedectomy (3/444 = 0.7%) and in none after stapedotomy (0/235 = 0%).

Table **28** shows the severe (20 dB, 20% discrimination) postoperative sensorineural hearing losses after stapedectomy and 0.4 mm stapedotomy. The statistical analysis (contingency Table with χ^2) demonstrates a highly significant difference (p < 0.01) in favor of stapedotomy for the hearing losses that occurred after 0.5 – 5 years. The number of hearing losses that occurred within 6 months after surgery is minimal in both groups, so that only a trend without statistical significance was found in favor of stapedotomy.

11.4 Revision Surgery

a) Causes of Failure

Between 1979 and 1989, 108 revisions were performed by the author because of failures of stapes surgery; 81/108 (= 75%) were revision stapedectomies, 27/108 (= 25%) were stapedotomies. Only 13 out of 81 stapedectomies (16%) and 9 out of 27 stapedotomies (33%) had been performed primarily in our department. Thirteen of the 27 revision stapedotomies were operated on with a 0.4-mm piston (seven with a wire Teflon piston and six with a Platinum Teflon Piston).

The time interval between first surgery and revision operation is shorter for stapedotomies than for stapedectomies (Table **29**). Fifty-one percent of the stapedectomies were reoperated on after more than 10 years, whereas 67% of the stapedotomies were seen in the first 4 years postoperatively.

The causes of failure in revision stapedectomies and stapedotomies are shown in Table **30**.

Table **28** Postoperative sensorineural hearing loss ($\geq$ 20 dB for 0.5 – 2 kHz, $\geq$ 20% speech discrimination

Type of surgery	0 – 0.5 years postop.		0.5 – 5 years postop.		Total	
	n	%	n	%	n	%
Stapedectomy (n = 444)	11	2.5	27	6.1	38	8.5
Stapedotomy (n = 233)	1	0.4	1	0.4	2	0.8

Fisch, U., Dillier, N. Technik und Spätresultate der Stapedotomie. HNO 1987;35:252 – 254.

Table **29** Time internal between first and revision surgery

Time interval	Stapedectomy n = 81	Stapedotomy n = 27
1 – 4 years	23 (28%)	18 (67%)
5 – 10 years	17 (21%)	7 (26%)
10 years	41 (51%)	2 (7%)

Table **30** Causes of failure in 108 revision operations

Pathology	Stapedectomy n = 81	Stapedotomy n = 27
Displaced prosthesis	21 (26%)	15 (56%)
Incus erosion	10 (12%)	4 (15%)
Malleus fixation	2 (3%)	6 (22%)
Obliterated oval window	42 (52%)	2 (7%)
Fistula	6 (7%)	– (–)
Total	81 (100)	27 (100)

The most frequent complication after stapedectomy was the reobliterated oval window (52% vs. 7% of the stapedotomies). A displaced prosthesis was most common after stapedotomy (56% vs. 26% in stapedecto-mies).

No fistulas were seen following a "true" stapedotomy, i. e. if the prosthesis was placed in an opening of the footplate that was only slightly larger than the piston. One of the fistulas was found after total stapedectomy with perichondrium interposition and a 0.8-mm wire Teflon piston. Another fistula was found after partial stapedectomy, perichondrium interposition, and a 0.6-mm wire Teflon piston.

b) Results

In a series of 50 cases operated on before 1980, revision surgery carried a significantly lower probability of success than a primary procedure (Table 31).

The results obtained in 94 revision operations performed between 1979 and 1989 are presented in Tables 32 and 33. The functional results of revision stapedotomy are superior to those obtained for revision stapedectomies. The reason for this difference must lie in the frequent presence of re-obliterated oval windows seen after stapedectomy. The most common failure of a 0.4-mm stapedotomy was related to prob-

Table **31** Hearing results in primary and revision surgery for otosclerosis

Air−bone gab (dB)	Primary operations (n = 189)		Revision operations (n = 50)		p
	n	%	n	%	
0−5	50/189	26.5	0/50	0	<0.01
0−10	106/189	56.1	9/50	18	<0.01
0−20	157/189	83.1	18/50	36	<0.01
0−30	181/189	95.8	24/50	48	<0.01
>30	8/189	4.2	7/50	14	<0.05

Table **32** Causes of failure and audiologic results of 81 revision stapedectomies (1979−1989)

Pathology	0 −10 dB	0−20 dB	0 −30 dB	> 30 dB
Displaced prosthesis (n = 26)	1 (4%)	10 (38%)	14 (54%)	12 (46%)
Incus erosion (n = 10)	1 (10%)	5 (50%)	9 (90%)	1 (10%)
Malleus fixation (n = 3)	2 (67%)	3 (100%)	3 (100%)	−
Obliterated oval window (n = 42)	3 (7%)	15 (36%)	26 (62%)	16 (38%)
Total (n = 81)	7 (9%)	33 (41%)	52 (64%)	29 (36%)

Table **33** Causes of failure and audiologic results of revision surgery after 0.4-mm stapedotomy (n = 13, 1979−1989)

Pathology	0 −10 dB	0−20 dB	0 −30 dB	− 30 dB
Displaced prosthesis (n = 6)	1	3	4	2
Incus erosion (n = 4)	1	4	4	−
Malleus fixation (n = 3)	1	3	3	−
Obliterated oval window (n = 0)	−	−	−	−
Total (n = 13)	3 (23%)	10 (77%)	11 (85%)	2 (15%)

lems of the prosthesis or of the incus. Systematic use of incus replacement and
stapedotomy (IRS) for the repair of failure
due to incus erosion, incus or malleus fixation, and a narrow oval window, has significantly contributed to improving the results
of revision surgery after stapes operations
(Table 34).

No deafness occurred in any of the 94 reoperated patients, even though 44 cases required opening of a reobliterated oval window.

Table **34**   Audiologic results 3 years after revision stapes surgery

Conductive deficit in dB	Incus replacement and stapedotomy n = 30	TORP n = 14
0–10	5 (17%)	– (–)
0–20	15 (50%)	4 (29%)
0–30	23 (77%)	8 (57%)
30	7 (23%)	6 (43%)

11.5 Results of Stapedectomy in the Presence of Unmeasurable Preoperative Hearing

Surgery in the presence of unmeasurable
hearing is performed whenever the well-ar-
ticulated speech of the patients indicates that
he or she is able to hear his or her own voice.
As shown in Table **35**, a hearing improvement permitting successful use of hearing
aids was obtained in 64% of the cases for 3
years or more. Surgery was more successful
in women than in men (p. < 0.05).

11.6 Results of Stapes Fixation without Otosclerosis

Stapes operations performed because of congenital fixation, congenital anomaly, or
anomaly of the facial nerve have given less
satisfactory results than those performed because of otosclerosis (Table **36**). On the other
hand, osteogenesis imperfecta as well as traumatic fixation of the stapes can be surgically
treated with a similar success rate as otosclerosis.

Table **35**   Results of stapedectomy in presence of unmeasurable * preoperative hearing (n = 23)

Sex	Age (years) ($\bar{x}$ + range)	Number of operated ears	Improved (3 years or more)	Hearing temporarily improved (2 months to 1 year)	Unchanged
Males n = 16	25–74 (54.8)	18*	9	3	6**
Females n = 7	40–71 (58.2)	7	7		–**
Total		25	16 (64%)	3 (12%)	6 (24%)
				Rim = 17/25 (68%) Oblit. = 8/25 (32%)	

*   2 cases with 50, respectively 56.6, bone conduction
** p < 0.05

Table **36** Stapes fixation without otosclerosis

| Type of pathology | n | Postoperative hearing | | | |
| | | Improved | | Unchanged | |
		n	%	n	%
Congenital stapes fixation	14	8/14	57	6/14	43
Congenital anomaly of stapes	6	3/6	50	3/6	50
Anomaly of facial nerve	3	2/3	66.6	1/3	33.3
Fragilitas ossea	2	2/2	100	0/2	0
Traumatic fixation of stapes	2	2/2	100	0/2	0
Total	27	17/27	63	10/27	37

12. Rules and Hints

- Operate on the worse ear first.
- Do not operate on the only hearing ear.
- Bilateral stapedectomy can be performed in adults at an interval of 1 year after the first successful surgery.
- Do not perform bilateral stapedectomy in children.
- Unilateral, low-tone sensorineural hearing losses may mimic a conductive hearing loss and lead to deafness if the stapes is removed.
- Do not operate on ears with tubal problems.
- Local anesthesia offers better surgical conditions than general anesthesia.
- Stapedotomy is less traumatic to the inner ear than stapedectomy.
- Stapedotomy performed before removing the stapedial arch avoids mobilization or fracture of the footplate.
- If you produce a larger opening than desired, close the vestibule with pressed perichondrium before placing the TPP.
- Avoid removing the superior edge of the footplate because of the frequent fibrous adhesions with the utricle in this area.
- Essential instruments for stapedotomy are the 0.2-mm, 90° footplate elevator, the crurotomy scissors, the 2.5-mm, 45° hook, and the straight alligator forceps.

- Stapedotomy with an intact stapes arch is only possible in the majority of cases if a 0.4-mm piston is used.
- The tip of the Teflon piston should penetrate 0.5 mm into the vestibule. The size of the prosthesis is criterion for a good result. The tip of the Teflon piston wire should not penetrate more than 0.5 mm into the vestibule.
- Saucerize the oval window niche with the diamond burr in obliterative cases until you uncover a blue area 0.4–0.5 mm in diameter. Clean the oval window niche of bone particles and remove the last bone shell with a 0.2-mm, 90° footplate elevator.
- Seal the stapedotomy opening with connective tissue, venous blood, and fibrin glue.
- Deafness is a tragedy, which, in most instances, is not an unavoidable complication of the operation, but the result of technical errors occurring during the performance of the operation.
- Take your time and be precise. Remember that for you, surgery is limited to 30–60 minutes, but the result will influence the patient for life.
- Remember that stapes surgery is a "one-go" procedure.
- If you encounter unexpected difficult con-

ditions, do not hesitate to close the wound and send the patient to someone with more experience. It takes more courage to step out from an operation than to continue it.

- Do not perform occasional stapedectomies.
- The surgical skills required for stapedotomy are superior to those needed for stapedectomy. This is not a disadvantage because the occasional stapes surgeon should be discouraged and the patients guided into more experienced hands. After a 0.4-mm stapedotomy, patients need more than 3 months to reach the final hearing result.
- The tympanomeatal flap should be elevated enough to expose the lateral process of the malleus and allow reliable assessment of the ossicular mobility.
- Incus replacement with stapedotomy (IRS) is the method of choice for the functional repair of malleus and/or incus fixation.
- There is less risk of inner ear damage with stapedotomy than with total stapedectomy.
- The prosthesis is less likely to migrate in stapedotomy than in stapedectomy.
- After stapedotomy there is no risk of lateral displacement of the oval window membrane in contrast to after stapedectomy.
- Use of the 0.4-mm TPP allows the systematic reversal of the classic steps of stapes surgery. The limited space between the stapes arch and facial nerve makes the consistent use of larger pistons impractical.
- If poor visualization dictates the need for canalplasty, it should be performed prior to elevation of the annulus from the sulcus to avoid contamination of the middle ear with irrigation while drilling.
- Visualization of the short process of the malleus, the tympanic segment of the facial nerve, and the pyramidal process is essential for proper performance of a stapedotomy.
- The inferior central two-thirds of the footplate is the safest place for the stapedotomy opening.
- The platinum loop of the prosthesis must be molded firmly to the incus for the best functional results. This is best achieved if the incudostapedial joint and the stapes arch are still intact.
- The intact stapes arch avoids undue movements of the piston within the vestibule while crimping the prosthesis.
- The platinum ribbon is malleable and conforms to the shape of the incus better than wire.
- The incudostapedial joint may be divided before placing the prosthesis if the stapes arch is left intact. This is done when there is doubt about the mobility of the malleus and of the incus.
- A tear in the tympanomeatal flap is best repaired with a pressed connective-tissue graft taken from the endaural incision.
- Manual perforators are better than electric drills because they allow the surgeon to "feel" the pressure of the tip of the instrument on the footplate.
- Scraping the mucosa around the stapedotomy opening favors taking of the connective tissue used to seal the opening into the vestibule.
- The laser beam is not superior to manual perforation of the footplate — particularly in the presence of a dehiscent and prominent facial nerve.
- Exact crimping of the prosthesis to the incus is more difficult than the creation of a calibrated hole through the footplate. The laser beam, unfortunately, cannot help fixate the loop of the prosthesis to the incus!

Appendix:
Instruments, Manufacturers, and Suppliers
of Microsurgical Equipment

In the following pages the interested reader will find data concerning the microsurgical equipment used for middle ear surgery in our institution. The instruments, sutures, and drugs mentioned in the book are also listed with the name and address of the manufacturer, the order number, and the page of citation in this book.

Manufacturers and Suppliers of Microsurgical Equipment

Microscope

Head	LEICA (Wild) AG Kanalstr. 21 8152 Glattbrugg Switzerland
Balanced contraves stand	Carl Zeiss Postfach 35/36 73447 Oberkochen Germany
Photo cameras (Contax)	Yashica AG Zürcherstr. 73 8800 Thalwil Switzerland
(Minolta)	Minolta Riedstr. 6 8953 Dietikon Switzerland
Video cameras	Hitachi
	Sony Baarerstr. 59 6300 Zug Switzerland
3D video	New Dimension Communication, Inc. R. Fabian, P.O. Box 4096 St. Charles, MO 63376 USA
Drape for microscope	Microtek Medical Ing. P.O. Box 2487 Columbus, MS 39701 USA

Drill

Motor	Bien-Air Länggasse 60 2504 Bienne Switzerland
Handpieces	Kavo Kaltenbach & Voigt International Steinbruchstr. 11 5200 Brugg Switzerland
Special handpiece for stapes surgery	Micro Mega SA Rue du Tunnel 5-12 25006 Besançon France
	Prodonta Micro-Mega Export Rue de la Mairie 3 1207 Geneva Switzerland
Burrs	Meisinger Kronprinzenstr. 5-11 40217 Düsseldorf Germany

Electrocautery

Bipolar	(Codman) Mediwar AG Birmensdorferstr. 360 8055 Zürich Switzerland
Unipolar	Mediwar AG Bernstr. 388 8953 Dietikon Switzerland
	Deltamed-Erbe AG Fröschenweidstr. 10 8404 Winterthur Switzerland

Microsurgical Instruments

(see also special list)

Leibinger (Fischer) GmbH
Bötzingerstr. 41
99111 Freiburg
Germany

Karl Storz GmbH & Co
Mittelstr. 8
78532 Tuttlingen
Germany

Bott AG, Arzt- und
Spitalbedarf
Genferstr. 2
8002 Zürich
Switzerland

Novimed Medizintechnik
Alte Landstr. 10
8955 Oetwil a.d.L.
Switzerland

J. Anklin AG
Baslerstr. 9
4102 Binningen
Switzerland

Middle Ear Prosthesis

Fisch Platinum-
Band Teflon
Piston
0.4 x 6.0
0.4 x 9.0

Xomed-Treace
6743 Southpoint Drive North
Jacksonville, FL 32216
USA

Fisch Spandrel II

Ionos Ossicle
5mm

Ionos, Med. Prod.
GmbH & Co

Ionos Neo-Mal-
leus

82229 Seefeld Obb.
Germany

Cialit (for preser-
vation of autol-
ogous and allo-
genous ossicles)

ASID Bonz & Sohn GmbH
85716 Lohhof b. München
Germany

Middle Ear Sheeting

Silastic

Laboratoire Perouse Implant
BP6-ZA D'Outreville
60540 Bornel
France

Ulrich AG
Mövenstr. 12
9015 St. Gallen
Switzerland

Gelfilm

Upjohn Company
Kalamazoo, MI 49001
USA

Diethelm & Co AG
Eggbühlstr. 14
8052 Zürich
Switzerland

Fibrin Glue

(Tissuecol)

Österreichisches Institut für
Hämoderivate GmbH
Immuno AG
Vienna
Austria

Immuno AG
Mühlebachstr. 38
8008 Zürich
Switzerland

Histoacryl-Glue

B. Braun Melsungen AG
Postfach 110 + 120
34212 Melsungen
Germany

Gelfoam
(Spongostan)

Novo Nordisk Pharma AG
8700 Küsnacht
Switzerland

Ferrosan A/S
2860 Soeborg
Denmark

Nerve Integrity
Monitor (Nim-2)

Xomed-Treace
6743 Southpoint Drive North
Jacksonville, FL 32216
USA

Dermatome

Downs Surgical Limited
Church Path
Mitcham Surrey CR4 3UE
Great Britain

Hausmann
Zürcherstr. 204
9014 St. Gallen
Switzerland

Cochlear Im-
plant (Nucleus)

Cochlear AG
Margarethenstr. 47
4053 Basel
Switzerland

List of Instruments, Sutures, and Drugs

	Manufacturer	Number	Page of citation
Alligator forceps, straight, large & fine	Leibinger (Fischer)	119 001	52, 53, 94, 123, 222, 223
Aluminum strip, malleable	Leibinger (Fischer)	118 215	22, 33, 128, 154, 169, 171
Array with electrode lead	Nucleus		204
Augmentin	Beecham		3, 188, 203
Bactrim	Hoffmann La Roche		3, 188, 203
Biopsy forceps (small)	Leibinger (Fischer)	119 060	24
Bipolar coagulation	Codeman	CMC 11	105, 229
Bipolar forceps, fine and large angulated tips 0.2 mm and 0.4 mm	Leibinger (Fischer)	017 682, 017 646	229

Burrs
– Sharp burrs (70 mm long)
  7.0 mm
  5.0 mm
  4.5 mm
  4.0 mm
  3.5 mm
  2.7 mm
  2.3 mm
  1.8 mm
  1.4 mm
  1.0 mm
 	
– Diamond burrs (70 mm long)
  7.0 mm
  5.0 mm
  4.0 mm
  3.1 mm
  2.3 mm
  1.8 mm
  1.4 mm
  1.0 mm
  0.8 mm
  0.6 mm
 	
– Diamond supercut (70 mm long)
  7.0 mm
  5.0 mm
  4.0 mm
  3.1 mm
  2.3 mm
  1.8 mm
	Meisinger	
		
		105 390
		105 386
		105 384
		105 382
		105 380
		105 372
		105 370
		105 368
		105 366
		105 364
		
		105 590
		105 586
		105 582
		105 578
		105 574
		105 572
		105 570
		105 568
		105 566
		105 562
		
		1504-70
		1504-50
		1504-40
		1504-31
		1504-23
		1504-18
			23–261

Caliper rod, 0.4 mm malleable	Leibinger (Fischer)	118 382	221, 241, 254
Catgut suture 2-0 Liga	B. Brown	07804	192, 193
Cochlear Implant: – Dummy array of receiver/stimulation with electrode lead Receiver/stimulation package – Implant template (metal) – Special claw for electrode insertion	 Nucleus Nucleus Nucleus	 Z 733 001 Z 730 003 Z 73 004 Z 73 005	 204 206 203 205
Crurotomy scissors	Leibinger (Fischer)	119 070, right 119 071, left	224, 239, 244
Curette (double)	Leibinger (Fischer)	118 542	218, 219

	Manufacturer	Number	Page of citation
Cutting block (stapedotomy)	Leibinger (Fischer)	119 300	77, 79, 220
Dermatom, Rosenberg skin grafting knives	Downs	430 916	138
Dexon 2-0 Liga	Davis & Geck	9010–51	207
Dressing forceps, fine	Leibinger (Fischer)	126 774, 126 766	28, 70, 75, 92, 102, 189, 233
Drill handpieces for surgery,			
– special	Micro-Mega, France	48E ORL	104
– straight	Kavo, Kaltenbach &Voigt Internat.	117 013	241, 247
– angled			
Ear speculum (black)	Leibinger (Fischer)	120 002	16, 121
Endaural raspatory	Leibinger (Fischer)	118 507	215
Endaural retractors	Leibinger (Fischer)	113 313	74, 88, 91, 124, 127, 131, 132, 215
Ethibond sutures, 3:0, 4:0	Ethicon	3:0 6663FS1 4:0 6683FS-2S	18, 193, 207, 227
Fascia scissors, curved	Leibinger (Fischer)	322 445	28
Fibrin glue, 0.5, 1.0, 2.0 ml	Immuno AG		53, 62, 77, 80, 159, 188, 226, 242, 244, 250, 259
Footplate elevator (Fisch), 90° 0.2 mm,	Leibinger (Fischer)		65, 81, 95, 161, 178, 226, 229, 241, 262
bent downwards		118 397	
bent upwards		118 399	
Gelfilm	Upjohn	0009-0297-01	2, 17, 83, 84, 86, 180, 181
Gelfoam 90x50x10 (Spongostan)	Ferrosan, Dänemark		17, 18, 26, 29, 30, 32, 34, 139, 141, 163, 217, 227, 259
Glass (Plastic)-Board 100 x 87 mm	Leibinger (Fischer)	50–1406	28, 76, 138
Histoacryl glue	Braun, Melsungen	105 005/2	125, 206
Hook, see microhook			
Ionocem (Cement)	Ionos	09832	105, 125
Joint knife	Leibinger (Fischer)	118 347/1	25, 224, 237
Key raspatory	Leibinger (Fischer)	119 506	20, 75, 92, 167, 229, 231, 232, 238, 239, 242
Lumbar drain	Cordis	910–109/ 910–110A	250
Malleus nipper	Leibinger (Fischer)	119 020	238
Manual perforators	Leibinger (Fischer)	118 393 (0.3 mm) 118 394 (0.4 mm) 118 395 (o.5 mm) 118 396 (0.6 mm)	52, 57, 77, 93, 221, 228, 239, 244, 245, 249, 254, 261, 262
Mastoid drain (Kaja drain)	Struba Gummi, 8039 Zürich	4x6x15	36, 106, 163
Mastoid raspatory	Leibinger (Fischer)	118 300 large 118 507 small	19, 187, 202

	Manufacturer	Number	Page of citation
Measuring rod, malleable (stapedotomy)	Leibinger (Fischer)	118 380	52, 59, 62, 77, 79, 89, 95, 220, 228, 231, 238, 241
Microraspatory (Fisch), universal	Leibinger (Fischer)	118 310 (right) 118 312 (left)	23, 47, 88, 128, 129, 131, 160, 168, 170, 173, 174, 216, 217
Microhook,	Leibinger (Fischer)		
0.5 mm, 45°		118 371	159, 179, 222, 243
0.5 mm, 90°		118 361	60
1.5 mm, 45°		118 373	6, 17, 27, 30, 32, 34, 46, 48, 65, 75, 77, 89, 91, 93, 95, 121, 122, 155, 178, 182, 185, 226, 237, 239, 257 16, 67, 71, 73, 229
1.5 mm, 90°		118 363	27, 28, 31, 52, 60, 67, 71, 73,
2.5 mm, 45°		118 374	89, 95, 181, 225, 237
Microsuction tubes			16, 31, 48, 60, 61, 66, 76, 93, 158, 159, 160, 181, 226, 241
(1.0 mm)	Leibinger (Fischer)	114 072/03	
(0.5 mm)	Leibinger (Fischer)	114 072/01	
(0.7 mm)	Leibinger (Fischer)	114 072/02	
olive	Leibinger (Fischer)	114 074	
Myringotomy knife	Leibinger (Fischer)	112 117	121
NIM-2 (Nerve Integrity Monitor)	Xomed-Treace		6, 137, 158, 159, 160, 172, 173, 203
Ossicle, Autograft			49, 72, 82, 89, 90, 92, 162
Ossicle, Ionomer (partial 5mm)	Ionos Med. Prod. GmbH	098 240	63, 72, 78, 79, 80, 82, 89, 91, 93, 113, 162
Otosporin	Wellcome		29, 34, 163, 226, 259
Prolene suture, 5:0	Ethicon	8661/FS2	141
Retroauricular retractor, rigid (black)	Leibinger (Fischer)	113 317/2	155
Retroauricular retractors, articulated (black)	Leibinger (Fischer)	118 455/2, 113 317/2	20, 33, 104, 135, 136, 137, 140, 141, 154, 155, 168, 169, 171, 172
Rongeur	Leibinger (Fischer)	118 140	179
Rubber bulb	Leibinger (Fischer)	110 917	36
Scalpel handle – for No. 11 blade	Storz	208 011	21, 66, 70, 168, 190, 216, 220
– for No. 15 blade	Storz	208 015	75, 92, 102, 167, 215
– for No. 4 blade	Leibinger (Fischer)	118 411	??
– for No. 7 blade, (16.5 cm long)	Leibinger (Fischer)	118 412	28
for No. 20 blade	Storz	208 010	28, 87, 138, 187
Scissors, straight (large)	Leibinger (Fischer)	320 446 118 437	138
Septal cartilage			101, 107
Septal raspatory	Leibinger (Fischer)	119 507	103, 105
Shea vein press	Storz	227 900	65, 233

	Manufacturer	Number	Page of citation
Silastic Sheeting, thickness 1 mm	Lab. Perouse, France	LP 502-1	83, 84, 99, 100, 107, 163, 180, 181, 182, 183
Skin hook	Leibinger (Fischer)	118 420	75, 92, 102, 191, 202
Small curved clamp	Leibinger (Fischer)	113 184	47, 62
Small curved clamp, modified for Ionomer Ossicle	Leibinger (Fischer)	113 184	49, 50
Spandrel II	Xomed-Treace	11-56295	54, 55, 56, 57, 58, 60, 61, 64, 66, 69, 70, 71, 73, 81, 82, 87, 89, 94, 95, 113, 260, 262
Stainless steel wire (0.0005 in) for CTW prosthesis	Storz	228 000	230, 231
Steristrips	3M		125
Suction irrigation	Leibinger (Fischer)	118 249 118 254/3 118 256/4	173, 174
Teflon Platinum-Band Piston, TPP 0.4 × 6 mm (Total length, including head, of 7 mm)	Xomed-Treace	11-56234	53, 64, 69, 77, 79, 80, 82, 93, 113, 214, 220, 222, 223, 232, 238, 239, 242, 244, 245, 246, 247, 249, 251, 252, 254, 256, 258
0.4 × 9 mm	Xomed-Treace	11-56238	51
Terracortril 10 g	Pfizer	551 683	163, 188, 227
Thermocautery	Erbe	ACC450	187
Tympanoplasty microscissors, curved	Leibinger (Fischer)	119 016 (left) 119 017 (right)	137
Tympanoplasty microscissors, straight, small and large	Leibinger (Fischer)	119 013 119 018	21, 27, 79, 127, 158, 184, 217, 224, 226, 230
Tympanoplasty scissors, curved	Leibinger (Fischer)	320 446	59, 88, 188, 191, 233, 237, 253
Ventilating tube T Goode Grommet Silicon	Xomed Treace	40 812 10-16 020	122, 123
Ventilating tubes (polyethylene)			121, 122
Vicryl suture, 4:0	Ethicon	V292ZFS2	139, 141
Watchmaker forceps	Leibinger (Fischer)	18 004	70, 137, 220, 226, 230, 231, 239
Wire bending die (Schuhknecht)	Leibinger (Fischer)	118 385	231
Wire scissors	Leibinger (Fischer)	118 388	57, 66, 231
Wound retractor (3–4 prongs)	Storz	800 403	167, 202

Index